CONCILIUM

concilium   1998/5

ILLNESS AND HEALING

Edited by

Louis-Marie Chauvet and
Miklós Tomka

SCM Press · London
Orbis Books · Maryknoll

Published by SCM Press, 9–17 St Albans Place, London N1
and by Orbis Books, Maryknoll, NY 10545

ISBN: 0 334 03051 x (UK)
ISBN: 1 57075 191 9 (USA)

Typeset at The Spartan Press Ltd, Lymington, Hants
Printed by Biddles Ltd, Guildford and King's Lynn

Concilium Published February, April, June, October, December.

Contents

Part III

Editorial

According to the World Health Organization, health is more than the absence of illness; it is a general well-being felt at a psychological and a moral level as well as at a physical level. Now while Western scientific medicine has made undoubted progress, as represented by the notable increase in average life expectation, it tends to put its remarkable techniques at the service of a very reduced conception of health, that of the body, and an often 'instrumentalized' body at that. That is why the first part of this issue of *Concilium* offers a series of reflections on this problem and seeks to illuminate it, referring on the one hand to much wider conceptions of illness and health in traditional societies, and on the other to attempts at 'alternative' practices in the current world of medicine in the West. It also relates illness to the social, economic and political malfunctions in our societies.

As is shown by the various articles in the second part, Christian faith has never been a stranger to problems of health. The basic reason for this lies at the heart of its message, the proclamation of a 'saviour' Jesus. Jesus manifested salvation not only by his words but also by his body, through his acts of healing and exorcism, to the point of the total gift of his person. We know that in pre-scientific cultures, the borderline between the physical and the psychological, the bodily and the spiritual, is ill-defined and always porous. Revelation clearly does not relate to cultural factors; thus it is quite legitimate to understand certain exorcisms practised by Jesus as healings, for example of epileptic crises. Revelation relates, rather, to two points. First of all it makes clear that the salvation to which human beings aspire can be integral and definitive only on two conditions: that it touches the very root of the human heart and that it is the work of God. In fact God alone can forgive sins (Mark 2.7); in doing this God offers an integral salvation. Apart from the famous episode of the forgiveness of the paralysed man in Mark 2.12, the expression 'forgiveness' of sins with which Luke sums up the realization of the promise (Luke 24.47; Acts 2.38) indicates the integral character of salvation, since it touches on that very root of evil-doing in the human heart which the Bible calls sin and which, before being an act, is a power (personalized in the figure of Satan) holding everyone under its yoke. Of course the expression 'forgiveness of sins' is not to be understood in an exclusive sense (sin, so in the end everything else does not matter very much), but in an inclusive sense: sin and *a fortiori* everything else (body; relationships; social, economic and political conditions). Then revelation involves the rejection of the idea that illness or infirmity are the fatal consequence of the sin of others (John 9.2–3).

In the footsteps and in the name of Jesus, its Lord, the church has not ceased to engage in symbolic actions of salvation encompassing the somatic, psychological and spiritual dimensions of the human being. The integration of these various dimensions is clearly a source of ambivalence. Several contributions in the second part show very well how, through its practices of healing, exorcism and protection against natural scourges throughout history, the church has been able to inculturate the Christian message; but they also show, without the need to adopt any theological perspective, the risks of the 'manipulation' of the divine power which have gone with these practices. The anointing of the sick, in the Middle Ages called extreme unction, is without doubt the best expression of this ambivalence, in that for the Catholic Church it is a properly sacramental act. This act was in fact the object of some more or less superstitious developments (which doubtless contributed to its progressive restriction to priests from the eighth century onwards), and in the interpretations which have been given to it down the ages it has almost constantly oscillated between physical effects and spiritual effects. However, we may ask whether this is not one of the finest expressions of Christian salvation, as is shown today by communal celebrations, provided that they have been well prepared and are carried out well. It is not unusual to see here a reconciliation of the sick at every level of their existence: with their sick bodies; with those around them on whom they accept that they are dependent; with the church, an unsuspected aspect of which they discover; and with God, at the end of a more or less lengthy process of rebellion against him. These benefits are not only psychological, moral, relational and spiritual but often have an effect on the body itself, which often feels better. Beyond doubt they can be read as the expression of what today is currently, and rightly, called a 'symbolic efficacy'. This is interpreted in faith as the effect of the 'grace of the Holy Spirit' (according to the sacramental word). The profound peace sensed by many sick on this occasion is a clear indication of the integral character of Christian salvation.

It is precisely this integral character that is sought by the numerous and varied new practices of healing which are attested (in part) in the third part of this issue. Here again, because of the very ambivalence of what is being investigated, the church must remain vigilant to possible false developments. But the church cannot take over this quest. That is particularly true of a continent like Africa, where the Christian notion of salvation and evil has been adopted in a way which fails to integrate a number of cultural values and traditional practices relating to illness and healing. To this must be added the various ills perceived as having been caused by white colonization: formerly political and now economic. In this context the so-called 'independent' churches, which are often 'syncretistic', easily 'win back' populations which do not find in the discourse and above all the practice of the great historical churches the 'salvation' that they seek. But even the Western countries today are experiencing a strong demand for healings of every kind: one need only mention the tremendous demands on diocesan exorcists, whom in some instances their dioceses have wanted for some decades to make technically redundant; the so-called 'charismatic' practices of healing in the ecclesial communities; or again the growing success of pilgrimages, first and foremost the pilgrimage to Lourdes. Similarly, we should note the growing importance, at least in France, of diocesan services arranged by the pastorate to the sick, and the various forms of spiritual support for Christians. All these symptoms indicate that the churches are faced with a real challenge. How can specifically Christian salvation be shown in demands which are often ambiguous?

Clearly this issue cannot cover all the aspects of the question. But at least it has attempted to sketch out the wide horizon and to show the urgency of rethinking the theology of salvation not only in its spiritual dimensions but also, in connection with these, in its corporal, social and cultural, economic and political dimensions. It has also, indeed above all, attempted to emphasize the interest that theologians are invited to show in the manifold practices of healing which flourish today. This is an enormous field of work!

Louis-Marie Chauvet
Miklós Tomka

Part I

Transitions in the Meaning of Health and Health Care: A First-World Perspective

Paul J. Philibert

Christians are accustomed from the Bible to think of illness and healing in terms that synthesize physical, mental and spiritual conditions. But the triumph of a scientific mentality in Western medicine in the past 150 years has progressively diminished the tendency to conceive of illness as a multi-faceted phenomenon and yielded to the habit of defining illness in exclusively physical terms.

What is health? It is the abundance of life and so involves a variety of aspects. Health is unimpaired physical integrity – the absence of wounds, fevers, weakness, pain or other types of distress. It implies strength and energy in the bodily organs, limbs and senses of a person and the experience of well-being and joy in living. To the degree that well-being is diminished or damaged, some aspect of illness is involved.

One quality of a fully alive person is peace of soul. Disease can damage the physical stability of life, thus ruining its quality and diminishing the integrity of health. Health is also modified by a person's experience of purpose and of community of purpose. One's mission in life is sustained and interpreted in terms of a network of others – family, colleagues, friends and community – who receive the contribution of one's work and generosity.

Such a vision of health helps us to articulate the meaning of illness, which is a destabilization of the forces of life. The sources of such destabilization can be war, violence, personal attack, contagion or injury. In human history, most generations have experienced the trauma of war and violence. In addition, famine, natural disasters and accidents lead to the disruption of physical and social well-being. Volcanoes, earthquakes, hurricanes or floods often mark the lives of whole communities.

Illness more commonly comes into ordinary lives through contagion with infectious diseases, cancer, heart ailments and abnormalities related to the endocrine, gastrointestinal, respiratory and the other functional systems of the body. History has marked some ages (the fourteenth and fifteenth centuries) with the horror of plague. Today we experience the equivalent of a plague phenomenon through widespread infection with HIV/AIDS illness unto death.

Beyond disease, illness is related to the gradual loss of powers characteristic of aging. Recent research has identified Alzheimer's disease and similar degenerative diseases characteristic of those moving into old age.

So there is no clear-cut criterion for illness. It is an analogical concept, realized in different phenomena in significantly different ways. Injury, pain, physical and social dysfunction are signs of a troubling condition of the person; but the condition can be caused by sources interior to the person or exterior, by ordinary degeneration of physical processes or by the intrusion into the body and its environment of infectious or debilitating influences.

The history of medicine shows us the escalation in recent centuries of our tendency to medicalize human experiences. The ancients accepted high infant mortality and a low life expectancy as facts of life. Many illnesses, such as stroke, heart trauma or cancer, were untreatable in previous centuries. Today, not only do such illnesses constitute the focus of a large majority of medical treatment, but the treatment of the terminally ill often aims at their continued survival even when the quality of life of the patient may be dubious (as if illness were an affront to scientific power).

Let us see if it is possible to make some reasonably accurate generalizations about the structure and biases of contemporary Western health care. What is the physician's focus of attention? What is the object of treatment? What is the vision of the patient as person? And how can these questions help us to understand our need to be more open to broader conceptions of healing and health?

The bias of Western scientific medicine

Consciously or unconsciously, sick people bring to their doctors their whole lives, that is, not only their concern about a symptom, pain, dysfunction or infection, but their concern about their families, their work, their continuity in a community of relations, and their anxiety about their ability to remain in or return to their personal and creative occupations. Even those fortunate enough to have easy access to a competent physician are often limited to a summary dialogue about their symptoms and medical history. To cite Sherwin Nuland, 'Today's physician has become a master of detached observation, but less of his patient than of his patient's tissues, fluids, and images as they can be studied by a variety of machines.'[1]

The assessment, diagnosis and treatment of the sick depend upon an immense structure of laboratory science that demands clinical distance from the person treated. Many physicians are more likely to attend to the reports of a radiologist or pathologist – read off graphs or a computer screen – than to the patient's description of complaints. Contemporary medicine is inclined to establish a relational distance between the caregiver and the patient, on the one hand, and to create a typology of disease from similar cases despite the uniqueness of the persons afflicted. The scientific discoveries that have allowed doctors to identify disease in a systematic way and treat it with confidence have also led to the rationalization of illness and the alienation of the patient.

In the 1860s and 1870s Pasteur, Lister and Koch had identified and explained the infection process of bacteria introduced as microscopic organisms into the fluids and tissues of the human body. The acceptance of germ theory, which allowed the detection of specific pathological elements in the blood or tissues of the patient, promoted the idea of distinct and single causes for specific sicknesses. One function of scientific assessment and diagnosis of the ill became and remains the analysis of the blood and urine of an ailing patient, a process designed to reveal the microbial presence of invading organisms within the body.

The nineteenth century also saw the introduction of three medical instruments which improved the accuracy of diagnosis. In 1819, the stethoscope was introduced for the auscultation of the heart and lungs; in 1830, an immense improvement in the lenses of the microscope gave physicians access to seeing smaller and more fragmentary parts of their patients; and in 1895, Roentgen discovered X-rays which allowed the viewing of organs inside the body without invading the body's tissues. New technological developments have opened even more amazing diagnostic windows onto the physical systems of the patient, including the CAT-scan, MRI and others. Scientific medicine now passes from surmise to certainty in the diagnosis of many diseases. But along with this objectivity comes a spirit of detachment from the person of the patient and from the particulars of the patient's complaints.

Another breakthrough in therapy began in the 1930s and continued during and after World War II. With the discovery of sulfa drugs, then of penicillin, and then of a series of major antibiotics, the medical establishment was able to treat effectively and destroy illness-producing viruses and bacteria that from time immemorial had been generally fatal for patients. The control of infection has been followed by the development of new forms of chemotherapy directed at the control or destruction of cancers in the human body. Some patients today live on a continuing regime of chemotherapy over a period of years as cancer patients. Chemical therapeutics make it possible for the patient to declare war on cancer – and in many lives that is the nature of the lived experience of illness. Chemotherapy, however, has also entered into reproductive science: there is now a chemotherapy designed to abort the foetus living in a woman's womb. Drug 'therapy' has become more than attacking an invading bacillus or virus; it has become a means to attack an 'invading foetus' as well.

Today these combined forces for diagnosis and therapy are harnessed to technology that allows for finer and finer specifications of surgical intervention. Procedures that were unthinkable in the last century – open heart surgery, organ transplants, surgery on the foetus *in utero*, for example – are now frequent and routine. We have come to anticipate an ongoing stream of scientific and technological breakthroughs that will represent the gradual realization of technical control over all the physical processes of human life.

The most dramatic medical frontier is perhaps the vast cooperative effort of research scientists called the Human Genome Project. At the present time, about 7,000 human genes have been identified out of an imagined 50,000 to 100,000 genes that distinguish the human species. Medical researchers dream of being able to detect genetically determined disabilities or illnesses, including various forms of cancer, in the patient or in prospective parents of children.

Today contemporary medicine, which began as compassionate therapy for wounded patients, frequently includes the exploitation of a utopian imagination by the physician or scientist as social architect. Medical technology may set aside philosophical or theological limits to the understanding of what is human. As Roy Branson and others have argued, medicine can operate as a substitute for religious belief and ritual. If 'science has replaced religion (narrowly defined) as the unifying focus of modern culture, then medicine is part of the central faith of our times'.[2]

Scientific fundamentalism, with medicine as the most salient practical example in society, sees itself as both the interpreter and manipulator of ultimate reality, standing guard over such questions as 'Who shall be born?' and 'Who shall be allowed to pass beyond life into death?'. The current fascination with cloning shows the tendency to apply to technical manipulation of the human body the principle 'whatever can be done, must be done'.

Challenges to medicine as ultimate reality

The international HIV/AIDS epidemic is calling into question the presumed technical omnipotence of therapeutic medicine. Twenty years of research have failed to produce a cure or an effective vaccine that can protect against HIV infection. At the same time, there have been outbreaks of new diseases that are virulent and lethal, the most familiar being the Ebola virus that has appeared in Africa in recent years. Infectious diseases long thought conquered, such as cholera, yellow fever and malaria, are reappearing in epidemic proportions again, often in strains that are resistant to previously successful treatments. In part, the problem may be due to overuse of antibiotic drugs for routine infections, leading to a diminished effectiveness of these drugs in those who have overused them. But viruses are also developing new strains that are resistant to familiar drug therapies.

Just as the only effective prevention of HIV infection at present is conscientious avoidance of sources of infection, so in other instances effective control of disease will depend upon scrupulous avoidance of contact with sources of infection. In a world of global travel and universal commercial contact, containment of disease to a local region of origin is increasingly difficult.

More positively, 'wellness' as a philosophy of care to assure good nutrition, aerobic exercise, regular periods of rest and withdrawal from work, moderation in the use of alcohol, and healthy relationships, is increasingly recognized as a vital part of health care. Many doctors request their patients to respond to extensive questionnaires which explore exactly these sorts of behaviour. It is now clear that prevention and healthy routines of nutrition and exercise are critical for good health.

Further, alternative forms of therapy are gaining respectability. Most major American cities have 'wellness clinics' that provide alternative therapies including nutrition counselling, acupuncture, and chiropractic medicine. The 'wellness' movement also advocates the benefits of meditation. The 'relaxation response' associated with meditation has been studied for some decades now and has been shown to be both beneficial to physical well-being and supportive of healing.[3] Recent studies show that religious belief and prayer are conducive to health and healing.[4] All of these dynamics lead beyond the single-cause diagnosis characteristic of a generation ago. Today many forces are leading people beyond the conception of illness as merely physical dysfunction and of medicine as purely surgical or pharmacological interventions.

Medicine as respect for life, realism about death

Powerful forces still resist an integral understanding of health and health care. North American society has elaborated a vast network of distractions to insulate people from the reality of their mortality. The popular culture diverts social consciousness from the reality of death through the glorification of sports, the illusions of advertising, the manipulation of sexual pleasure as a consumer object, and the progressive insinuation of suicide and mercy killing into public acceptance. Philip Keane has written,

> If we try to deny the reality of death, we are likely to make every conceivable attempt to prevent death, even when such efforts only serve to prolong dying and suffering . . .; if we adopt the false assumption that we can make everyone's death easy, we run the risk of failing to provide life-sustaining treatments which people justly deserve, or even the risk of adopting mercy killing as a means of easy social management of health care delivery.[5]

We are obviously at a cultural and ethical crossroad world-wide. In the First World, medicine has imagined health as the management of physical systems, seeking not only to vanquish sources of disease or to repair failing limbs and organs, but also to help parents to produce ideal progeny (or defend themselves against less than ideal offspring). This 'scientific' vision of medicine has come up against serious restraints – the escalating costs of technologically sophisticated treatments, the disenfranchisement of the poor, and the growing impersonalism of the relation between healer and patient.

Writers like Sherwin Nuland and Herbert Benson are proposing a distinction between the science of curing disease and the art of healing the patient's illness. In this sense, to *cure* is to treat diseased organs and tissues, looking not at the person but the pathology. On the other hand, to *heal* is to render patients at ease as whole persons within the structure of their spiritual world-view, their families, and their culture. Healing is largely about restoration that begins inside the patient.[6]

Will this crossroad in medicine lead to a new kind of synthesis, just as technical advances in the past have transformed the healing profession? Surely we will not abandon the scientific advances that are like miracles in the treatment of what in previous centuries were fatal and hopeless conditions. But as we acknowledge the need for a renewed vision of health care, we face a decisive moment where the spirituality of patients, their relationships and their purpose in life have come to possess a relevance frequently forgotten over the two centuries of medical miracles that have brought us to today.

How can these two streams merge? Perhaps the accounts that follow will amplify our understanding of the possibilities.

Notes

1. Sherwin B. Nuland, 'Doctors and Deities', *The New Republic*, 13 October 1997, 33.

2. Roy Branson, 'The Secularization of American Medicine', in S. E. Lammers and A. Verhey (eds.), *On Moral Medicine: Theological Perspectives in Medical Ethics*, Grand Rapids 1987, 25.

3. Herbert Benson, *The Relaxation Response*, New York 1975; *Your Maximum Mind*, New York 1989; *Timeless Healing: The Power and Biology of Belief*, with Marge Stark, New York 1996.

4. Keven Culligan, OCD, 'Spirituality and Healing in Medicine', *America* 175 5, August 1996, 17–21; K. Culligan, 'Are We Wired for God?', *America* 176 9, March 1997, 23–4.

5. Philip S. Keane, SS, *Health Care Reform: A Catholic View*, Mahwah, NJ 1993, 64.

6. See Nuland, 'Doctors and Deities' (n. 1); also Herbert Benson, *The Wellness Book: The Comprehensive Guide to Maintaining Health and Treating Stress-Related Illness*, New York 1993.

The Longevity of the Practice of Traditional Care

Eric de Rosny

Do we have to reserve the term 'scientific' for official medicine and 'traditional' for other practices of care? As if science did not have its traditions and popular cultures, from which other forms of therapy, their rigour and their logic, emerged! However, a kind of demarcation line has come to be drawn in people's minds between a so-called 'scientific' medicine, which arose in the West, which has become established all over the world and which for short I shall call 'hospital medicine', and a popular approach to medicine, common to the majority of cultures, which has been called 'traditional' to distinguish it from the former.[1] Even if the terminology is questionable, there is some justification for this contrast between planetary medicine and universal medical practices. As proof, here is an anecdote.

Quasi-universal practices

In 1982 I was invited to Nuremberg to a congress on the practice of the 'healers' whom the World Health Organization calls 'tradi-practitioners'; there, thanks to the German organizers, I found myself among researchers from all over the world, from Korea to Peru and from South Africa to Germany, via Cameroon, where I live. Each had an hour to present a film or slides, or simply to speak to the audience. No time was reserved for questions and discussions. There was great frustration among these specialists. Was this because of the inexperience of the organizers? I doubt it. It was rather a feeling on their part of what was going to happen.

From the second day on it became clear that we almost all used the same terminology and showed traditional treatments which manifestly obeyed the same rules, sometimes even with the same key words. So much so that we no longer had any questions to ask. For example, I was surprised when, on questioning an old German healer in private, he gave me, word for word, the reply that I had obtained from an equally venerable healer whom I met on the coast of Cameroon. 'When a visitor comes towards you, how do you know if you could cure him or not?' 'My body tells me,' they replied, each in his own language and a long way from one another. Despite the distance and the variety of cultures, there is a common practice which allows me, perhaps unduly, to generalize the result of my researches based solely on Africa.

During this congress three main features emerged as naturally the majority of the experiences which all the researchers presented: these are essentially *sacred* medical practices; all of them have a *social* dimension; and they are based on the *power* of the person giving the treatment. Is it a coincidence if these are precisely the features which cannot be found, or can only be found to a much less marked degree, in hospital medicine? This is not fortuitous and can be explained. On the one hand, these researchers, most of them trained in Western culture, could not proceed otherwise than by comparison with their original medicine, even if they were not always aware of this: the confrontation is certainly evocative, but it tended to exaggerate the differences. On the other hand the very history of medicine has been concerned with opening up the gap; as Jean-Paul Lévy remarks, 'the history of hospital medicine is to a great degree that of the progressive replacement of healers by medicine, with the rationalization of the body and illness . . . a process which is still far from coming to an end, supposing that it ever does'.[2] One doubts that.

The example of Cameroon

I could easily have found these characteristic features of traditional practice in around forty practitioners from the Cameroon coast whose techniques I studied at that time. Here is an illustration.

A sacral context. One person whom I had had to advise to seek 'indigenous' care came back to see me earlier than expected: 'This healer keeps saying that it is God who cures, not him! So why not send me straight to God?' Leaving aside the real reasons which made him give up the treatment, I would simply note what is significant in his reaction: for their success the practitioners do not depend on their art; they regard themselves as working for a hierarchy of invisible powers – ancestors, deities and God himself. This is so much the case that they do not claim the title 'healer' which they are usually given in French. In contrast to this sacral vision of sickness and healing, hospital medicine sees itself as essentially 'secular' and depending on the competence of the hospital doctors.

A social dimension. In the course of a treatment that was to last all night, another tradi-practitioner, who was called 'nganga' in Bantu, suddenly uttered a little phrase which is highly significant for the subject with which we are concerned. As always, the young sick girl whom he was looking after was accompanied by her family. But some members of this family had clearly had a few drinks and their euphoria affected the course of the treatment. In agitation, the nganga came up to them and said, 'Can't you see that you're the ones I am caring for through your daughter?' Hospital medicine tends to centre primarily on the individual, the organic body of the individual, even a single member of this body.

The exercise of a power. Popular practice is based on the 'power' of the practitioner considered as a 'gift'. It is not natural but received, whereas medicine is based on 'knowledge' acquired at the university. This distinction is sometimes a source of misunderstandings between researchers or ethnologists and those whose practices they study. The former come with the intention of acquiring knowledge, while the latter can think that their visitors want to acquire a 'power' among them. In some cases, moreover, they are ready to confer this power. For a while I myself have been the object of this scorn before benefiting from it.[3]

This degree of opposition between the two practices certainly should not be emphasized more at this level. It is evident, for example, that a traditional practitioner follows an apprenticeship and that by virtue of this he too acquires a *knowledge*, even if he gives the impression of attaching little importance to it compared to the *power* which he receives from his ancestors. A hospital doctor sees himself given real *power* in the eyes of his patients and can often use it to give them confidence. In this way a certain quality of relationship develops between the carer and those being cared for which cultural differences will not remove, however deep they may be. Nevertheless, there are differences between the two practices which the culturalist approach is not enough to justify and which relate to anthropology. Anthropology, also called 'the study of the logic of behaviour', makes it possible to have a better grasp of the original traditional therapeutic practices as compared to hospital medicine, over and above historical and cultural factors.

Practices which seek to be global

Who is the sick person? He or she is essentially the member of a family. In the sick bay, this is not just an isolated individual, visibly spread out on a mat; in reality the whole family is sick. The patient is the living sign of an ill which affects this family of which he or she is an integral part, to the degree that the invalid identifies with the family and the family recognizes itself in the invalid. What is usually called *illness* at hospital would be better translated *symptom*, the symptom of an evil which is gnawing at the group. Ultimately the illness of an individual becomes the occasion, I would dare to say the pretext, for recognizing the conflictual situation of the family. The task of this mediator, who is the soothsayer-practitioner, thus consists in discovering or allowing the family to discover the internal evil which is undermining its unity. He will care for the organic ailment of his patient with his herbs and his barks, but at the same time he will set out to discover and reveal to those around the patient, with more or less tact depending on his skill, the human cause of the ailments, namely the maleficent sorcery which is undermining them. It is up to them, by meetings or a discussion, to re-establish its threatened unity. As Peter Geschiere rightly points out:

> Even in modern contexts, sorcery almost always seems to arise from within the family. That is why it is an omnipresent and almost inescapable threat. In some respects sorcery is the dark side of kinship; it is a reckoning with the terrifying fact that there is jealousy, and thus aggression, within the family, where only confidence and solidarity should reign.[4]

Family bonds cannot be reduced to the visible family but extend to the dead, who include the founders of the line or eminent people to whom the status of ancestors is given. The practitioner addresses the latter to find the energy necessary for the care. But some among these dead people are the cause of the disorders in the family and more particularly of the evil from which one of its members is suffering. They have good reason for that, the soothsayer reveals, when the family is not run well and, most frequently, has failed to honour its dead as custom requires. In the most serious cases they show this in the sick bay by taking possession of the sick person or one of those around him or her, who progressively loses awareness of his or her identity. The person goes into a trance, under the control of the practitioner, and the dead man who for the moment inhabits the person delivers his accusation. This is a spectacular liturgy, doubtless the finest and most significant expression of the traditional religions.[5]

In a similar context, in which the sickness is a social affair, we can understand the rites having a therapeutic aim. They make it possible to mobilize the group concerned through a language which everyone understands without saying a word, which involves the body together with the objects representing the world around in miniature. The rite takes place where the visible and the invisible meet, as a manifestation of the corporal and relational dimensions of the human being. As François Laplantine points out, 'the rituals are not survivals of obscurantism, but the very expression of a constitutive dimension of illness and medical practice itself: its social relationship'.[6] We owe to Claude Lévi-Strauss a famous expression already existing in the Christian theology of the sacraments and here applied to health, namely that of the 'symbolic efficacy' of the rites.

Who is the sick person? The sick person is his or her own body for the moment duplicated. In the sick bay, not only *the visible body* of the sick person lying on the mat is affected, but the whole person. Before your eyes you have a carnal envelope, the appearance of a human being, while this person's double, the vital principle, the *invisible* dimension of the body which escapes ordinary eyes, is separated from it. Illness – once again the symptom of a lack of family union – resides in this dislocation of the two parts of the body. The analysis of his state of health which one of these patients made to me in Douala is significant:

> The day I arrived at the practitioner's my body felt empty. But after two days I began to feel that I was returning to myself. In other words, I was beginning to understand how my body was. Then I went on to the major treatment. There he said that the treatment was to make my double (*edi*) return so that I could see that my body had returned. It was then, after my double had returned, that I began to understand my life myself, how it was going on. But I still suffer a little from stomach-ache.

In this perspective, healing coincides with the return of the invisible body to its mould, which is the visible body, through the care of the practitioner.

This representation of illness and healing is thus based on a different conception of the human being from that which governs the medical strategy of hospitals. There the human being is essentially a body which duplicates itself; here it is a soul and a body. At the hospital everything goes on as if only the (visible) body were being looked after and the (invisible) soul were being left to the care of the churches. This demarcation based on the two elements in the human being, which today is very clear, derives from the historical compromise that the spiritual and temporal powers have progressively developed in the West, basing themselves on a hylomorphic view of human beings drawn from Greek philosophy. We should note in passing that the Bible offers a view of the human being closer to the anthropology underlying traditional practices than that of Hellenism.[7]

However, we have to ask whether there is in fact a difference between the 'invisible body' of the traditions with which we are concerned and the 'invisible soul' of the Greeks. This question needs to be noted since it is not without consequences for therapeutic treatment. The 'invisible' body is always considered as *material*, since the initiated who are given a double view have senses to see it, while the soul of the Greeks is conceived as *immaterial* and beyond the human gaze. So in the sick bay the notion of immateriality makes no sense; this avoids any dichotomy at this level, ensures easier communication between the different sectors of individual and social life, and gives the traditional practices this global aspect which is recognized, opposing it to the fragmented notion of medicine. Here we have two rational conceptions of the human being, which lead to two differentiated practices.

Conclusion. For the sake of clarity, this account has contrasted two systems which divide the world of health care: one is symbolized by the hospital and the other by ancient medicinal practices, which are still used today. Readers have doubtless noted that the term 'medicine' has not been used to characterize the latter. However, it is customary to speak of 'traditional medicines' alongside scientific medicine. But the parallel is not so simple. The panorama of health today is occupied by a quantity of forms of care deriving from medicine – parallel, alternative medicine – which the traditions – clairvoyance, healing practices, charlatanism – represent, to use Jean Benoist's happy phrase, as a 'constellation of recourse'.[8] Not to mention here the many forms of prayer for healing which are practised by the churches or come from them. So it is perhaps better to restrict the term medicine to public health, so as not to add to the existing confusion. At a time when the quest for healing is becoming a mark of civilization and sometimes an obsession, we find three groups devoted to health: medicine proper, a great diversity of syncretistic practices and the heritage of ancestral traditions. These last, which are an issue here, represent a totality which keeps its homogeneity, its identity and a degree of efficacy. Hence their amazing longevity.

Translated by John Bowden

Notes

1. To add to the confusion of the vocabulary, the term 'traditional' is often attached in the West to hospital medicine, to distinguish it from the new forms of so-called parallel or alternative therapies.

2. J. P. Levy, *Le pouvoir de guérir: une histoire de l'idée de maladie*, Paris 1991, 98.

3. E. de Rosny, *Les yeux de ma chèvre, sur les pas des maitres de la nuit*, Paris 1981.

4. P. Geschiere, *Sorcellerie et politique en Afrique*, Paris 1995, 18.

5. In East Asia it is the shaman who goes into a trance and not the patient. For this distinction see L. de Heusch, *Pourquoi l'épouser*, Paris 1971.

6. F. Laplantine, *Anthropologie de la maladie*, Paris 1986, 350.

7. P. Beauchamp, *Psaumes nuit et jour*, Paris 1980, 54, 'The prayer of the body'.

8. J. Benoist, *Anthropologie medicale et Société Créole*, Paris 1993, 85.

The Criticism of Scientific Medicine and the Attractiveness of Western 'Alternative' Methods of Healing

Michael Nüchtern

The therapeutic landscape is changing. So-called alternative methods of healing are increasingly gaining popularity alongside scientific medicine. A wealth of therapeutic ways are opening up, particularly in cases of chronic suffering, disturbed states and indeed the most severe illnesses: bleeding and primal cries, homeopathy and dancing, reincarnation therapy and acupuncture, kinesiology and aromatherapy, fresh cells and ayurveda . . . Granted there has always been some plurality in ways of dealing with health and illness, but the impression that today the variety in the therapeutic landscape is particularly great may well be correct.

To put it very simply, four large and different regions in the therapeutic landscape can be identified.

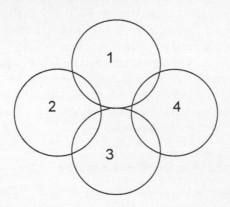

1. Exposing oneself to the stimulus of light, air and water to the right degree, breathing and moving correctly, eating sensibly, living in biological rhythms, i.e. in the sequence of sleeping and waking, stress and relaxation, is part of a consciously healthy life-style. Nowadays 'healthy living' orientated on experience is also offered professionally and in a focussed way by groups and organizations which are by no means just therapeutic, and are presented in a great variety of packages. Fasting cures, jogging, time-management and relaxation courses are current examples of this growth area. The old dietetics lives on here to a large degree, considerably transformed, in the form of Eastern physical exercises and esoteric experience of the body. Here 'health' is experienced and learned.

2. Family doctors of the old school combine elements of the first region with the second, the sphere of medicine on a scientific basis. Here illnesses which can be scientifically examined are diagnosed and therapy is provided.

3. The manifold supplements to and extensions of scientific medicine through ancient systems of medicine from foreign lands or new procedures from special sources of knowledge are to be located in a further region. As a result of the international exchange of information, elements of other cultures are being appropriated in the prosperous 'Western societies' as colonial goods and are uncontemporaneously contemporaneous. Their fascination, and individual experiences, lead patients and indeed doctors to seek supplementary ways to healing in Chinese, homeopathic, Indian, African or other therapies. Here the differences between somatic therapy and psychotherapy become blurred.

4. The supplementation can go so far that scientific medicine is deliberately replaced by other methods, often of a magical kind. Some elements of the first region can appear in this fourth region, when for example it is claimed that all illness can be prevented or healed by the choice of food or particular physical exercises.

In describing the criticism of scientific medicine expressed in the rise of alternative methods of healing we must first of all consider the characteristics of this medicine. However, the boom in alternative medicine is not just grounded in the repudiation of so-called 'classical medicine'; it is a cultural phenomenon.[1]

I. The character of scientific medicine

When I was sick as a child, the doctor used to ask, 'Where does it hurt?' This question was reassuring; it showed that now the expert had come and he could deal with the trouble, find its cause and thus remove it. On the other hand, my answer to the question 'It hurts here' wasn't my first and immediate reaction to being ill. This was better put in the words, 'I feel weak, I'm anxious, I hurt.' There wasn't room for the 'I' in an answer to the doctor's question. The nature of the question ruled it out. Insignificant though the type of question may appear, the nature of scientific medicine is reflected in it: the 'I', how the patient feels, is less interesting than the objective state of things. Doctors are the ones who time and again have drawn attention to this.'[1]

The classic procedure of the doctor in making a diagnosis is a detailed narrowing down and orientation. In so doing the doctor moves away from the immediate feelings of the sick person and concentrates on the measurable causes of the symptoms. In medicine, too, scientific thought and action begin with an isolation of phenomena from an overall context. In moving from the concrete totality of a feeling person to the elements and causes, in measuring and collecting numerical values in the medical investigation, Bacon's formula *dissecare naturam* (dissect nature) recurs. The concentration on numbers and findings reflects Descartes' conviction that having a physical reality at one's disposal amounted to the control of the reality itself. Because – according to a remark by Max Planck – the real is what can be measured, the scientific doctor is more interested in the findings than in the feelings, the objective than the subjective. In 1865 one of the fathers of modern physiology described the consequences of this world-view for the image of the human being very clearly: 'The living organism is only a marvellous machine, equipped with the most wonderful and complicated . . . mechanisms.'[2]

The successes of medicine in individual instances and in certain illnesses make this view plausible. But at the same time they alienate the patients from their bodies and from their health.

– whether by understanding themselves as machines and coming to think that findings are more important than feelings (when asked how he is, the patient in the clinic remarks that his blood pressure is better), – or often criminally underestimating their own power and the need to collaborate in health and sickness.

The 'view' given by scientific medicine teaches us to see where earlier there was unenlightened darkness. But it sees only a section, a realm of reality: what can be measured and objectified. Through the progress of medicine, on the other hand it suggests that everything belongs in this sphere. What cannot be fitted into a frame and measured and objectified runs the risk of being regarded as unreal: individual and unique, the therapeutic dimension of relationships and encounters.

The oncologist Harald Theim has shown that with the progressive objectification in medicine, specialization and advancing technology, the totality of its claim also grows:

> The better modern medicine can fulfil the expectations of health, the more it seems to be a power on which one can become dependent. On the one hand this development follows the development of the Baconian principle from the beginning of scientific practice that knowledge is power – this immense, accumulated, expanded, specialized, objectified knowledge of illness and the (clearly lesser) knowledge of the possibilities of healing. On the other hand the subjective ignorance about his own fate of the individual hungry for health has become the strong root of dependence and results in the powerful position of modern medicine, which could elevate health to be the supreme norm.[3]

Modern medicine is secular self-understanding plus science.

Medicine has directed its searchlight on more and more spheres of life – completely to the good. At the same time the light has become stronger and stronger, so that more has become possible and can be done. Human life can be artificially generated and manipulated; it can be sustained in premature babies outside the womb at an increasingly early stage. Under the conditions of intensive medicine, dying has changed from something that has to be accepted to a process that can be directed: lengthened or shortened. It is always the case that where there was once fate or nature, there is now civilization, i.e. medical action or lack of action.

It can be observed that the competence of medicine and therapy has extended to more and more phenomena in life: to insomnia, beauty, a capacity for guilt, mourning, old age, difficulties in learning, loving and living, and needs of every kind, and also to the capacity to work, compensation for handicap and much else. The concept of illness has also logically extended in parallel to the extension of the sphere of medical competence. With some justification it includes psychological, social and spiritual factors. The factors involved do not limit the power of medicine but extend it. Medicinalization is not good for all these phenomena in life. 'Illnesses' as such are 'invented' from social and cultural causes.[4] Striking features like the position of teeth and the size of noses are assessed and treated as illnesses. The total claim of medicine is matched by a total expectation on the part of the public that medicine can assess and remedy needs and heal damage. The annual increase in the

seamlessly into religious forms. 'I look for my own therapy' is the new motto.

Because of its reference to questions of meaning, not only will the therapeutic landscape grow wider and larger, but the therapeutic offers will so to speak go deeper and deeper. They relate to a variety of experiences of alienation. So the offers of alternative therapies contain an abundance of code words for unalienated life, a whole world: nature, centre, self, energy, creative potential, simple.

As long as everyday life runs in an orderly way the question of the meaning of life is not raised. This question emerges only when the everyday world is shattered. It appears that situations by which the everyday world is threatened are now being experienced, if not more frequently, at any rate more persistently than before. The more unsatisfying everyday life is, the more it is filled with crises, the more a longing arises for a new horizon for life which embraces the wealth of individual experiences and integrates them. Such a horizon is no longer generally available. It has to be found or adopted by individuals – however and wherever. A wide range of aids and helpers is available here. The realm of therapy offers means of coping with individual crises in a time when there is a sense of total crisis. The therapy scene offers itself as a fast track towards the project of one's own life – with what is offered there a person can unfold and develop individually – and an ambulance for those victims who have not reconciled the lofty goal of their own life with their everyday life in an alienated world and nature. The modern Western process of individualization with its secret pressure towards self-development conducts the gentle melodies of the psycho-scene in a hard and hidden way; the magic tones of the scene lure precisely those who long for the alternatives to modernity. To exaggerate: the therapy scene brings healing, but to a degree also the illness which it claims to heal. It propagates a norm and then promises to fulfil it: the norm of the 'whole', fully-developed, positive life, which can leave and has left suffering and negativity far behind it.

No wonder that the offers of the therapy scene are interwoven with esoteric, magical and religious ideas! Very often they communicate, directly or indirectly, a 'vision' of life and the world which can no longer be taken for granted elsewhere. And they have to do that because they relate to the experiences of deficiency already mentioned:

The high value attached to vitality and health,
 – the lack of clarity in the concepts of health and illness,
 – the discontent with science, technology and classical medicine,

- the pressure towards individualization and
- the longing for meaning with an increase in experiences of contingency.

All these mean that in particular the spheres of the enlargements or extensions of scientific medicine and the replacement of scientific ways of dealing with health and illness (see 3 and 4 above), and the spheres of training the body and life-style, are specific areas of growth (see 1 above). Therapy – understood as an evolving improvement and qualitative enhancement of life and possibilities in life – here becomes the key concept in the understanding of life generally. Here life always appears less simple, but open to shaping and change. If in scientific medicine the body is regarded as a machine capable of improvement, in other therapies the self is the unity which is capable of enhanced experience.

The notion of development with its impulse towards an enhancement and improvement of quality is not false. For Christians, it can be grounded and assessed in terms of the task given by creation; ethically, it can be grounded in the sense of responsibility. It would be fatal to abandon it. But where there is light there is also shade. Evolutionary thought becomes problematical where it absolutizes itself, and the balance between task and the givenness of life is no longer preserved. For then life no longer has dignity and value intrinsically, but only to the degree that it is capable of improvement and an enhancement of experience. Here the notion of euthanasia can gain influence as the dark brother of the developmental world-view.

III. Therapy as a partial or total goal: healing and wholeness

If my theses about the reasons for the extension of the sphere of therapy are correct, then parts of the therapy market are not just concerned with health and sickness in the narrower sense but potentially also with meaning in life. The attraction and seduction of what is on offer lie precisely in this great claim; so do the problems. The somewhat hazy goals are no longer the removal of the defect of a particular illness but the harmonization, development, transformation of the whole person: inward maturity, happiness and satisfaction. If what is offered promises such utopian goals as happiness and harmony, it can be dangerous. It threatens the certainties of given, everyday life for the sake of uncertain goals. The happiness and the successes in therapy promised apparently justify not only immense costs but in some circumstances also comprehensive control of life and changes in life. If the therapist belongs to a school with utopian goals, he will immediately assess all those seeking advice as in need of therapy; and because of the promises held out by therapy, these will feel themselves in need of therapy (thus H. Hemminger). In such a therapy, the chances of ever becoming 'healthy' are slim. By contrast, a decisive characteristic of a trustworthy therapy is not the promise of a utopian wholeness but a limited, realistic offer which can be checked. Not only in politics but also in the case of the individual the maxim holds that those who want to attain in immanence what is reserved for transcendence will do violence to human dignity and freedom.

The strength of the alternative approaches which replace and extend scientific medicine, their orientation on totality, is at the same time their problem. If an increasing number of spheres of life fall under the competence of a trainer or therapist, there is a danger of dependence and damage because the therapist or trainer has no competence in the manifold spheres of life. Professionalization, where it relates to such comprehensive goals as learning to live, carries with it the danger of producing dependent clients. Over against an extension of the problems for which therapists, advisers and trainers claim competence, an art of distinction needs to be practised which is guided by the question what the goal of therapy can realistically be. What seems to me to be needed today is not some extended therapy and healing art, but an ethically limited medicine.

The quantitative and qualitative extension of the sphere of therapy and the way in which it has come to be mixed up with experience and religion no longer automatically brings health; as a side-effect it brings new risks and dangers. What is to be done? First, perhaps, we need the simple perception that health and meaning in life cannot be produced technically; they cannot be achieved just like that. The risks in life cannot be transformed into complete certainty. Finitude and fragmentariness are part of life, and so are illness and dying. That is not a scientific but a religious statement. 'You are on earth and God is in heaven,' we read in the book of Ecclesiastes (5.1).

Theology and religion know how to distinguish healing and wholeness. There can be wholeness where there is no healing. There can be healing where there is no wholeness. Wholeness is hidden – sometimes under its opposite; healing can always be demonstrated. Wholeness is a special reality in relationship, healing a general possibility. So healing is potentially ubiquitous, possible everywhere, whereas wholeness is not possible everywhere but is real in a particular relationship. Healing can be done actively, wholeness is experienced passively. Through healing the patient becomes an agent; by contrast, even for the most active, wholeness involves being a 'patient'. The experience of wholeness interrupts everyday experiences; healing improves them and enhances them. In the Christian understanding, in the sphere of creation where human beings are fellow workers with God, wholeness belongs in the sphere of redemption, which is still to come but which can be experienced in parable form in the reality of creation – in becoming healthy and in enduring illness (II Cor. 12.9).[10]

Translated by John Bowden

Notes

1. E.g. K. Köhle and P. Joraschky, in Thure von Uexküll (ed.), *Psychosomatische Medizin*, Munich 1990, 415ff., referring above all to the works of Viktor von Weizsäcker.

2. Quoted from Heinrich Schipperges, *Moderne Medizin im Spiegel der Geschichte*, Stuttgart 1970, 232.

3. 'Entwicklungstendenzen der Medizin', in *Religion und Gesundheit*, Herrenalber Texte 85, 1986, 54.

4. Cf. Dieter Lenzen, *Krankheit als Erfindung*, Frankfurt 1991.

5. For more detail see E. Nüchtern, *Was Alternativmedizin populär macht*, EZW-Texte 139, 1998.

6. 'The history of medicine shows that a system of ideas about healing is not accepted by parts of the population primarily because of its clinical successes but because of the power of conviction, the plausibility of its basic ideas. If the ideas carry conviction, then successes in healing which are aimed at in the course of a therapy will be interpreted as consequences of the therapy', P. U. Unschuld, 'Schulmedizin und Therapie Freiheit', *Kursbuch* 119, 1995, 129.

7. Cf. E. Nüchtern, 'Alternativmedizin – eine romantische Bewegung', *Münchner Medizinischer Wochenschrift* 139, 1997.

8. *Risikogesellschaft. Auf dem Weg in eine andere Moderne*, Frankfurt 1986, 206.

9. *Die andere Realität* 2, 1993, 8.

10. For more details see M. Nüchtern, *Medizin, Magie, Moral*, Stuttgart 1995; id., *Was heilen kann*, Göttingen 1994.

Illness, Healing and Health: Economic, Legal and Social Dimensions

Lars Thielmann

From antiquity to the nineteenth century people experienced illness predominantly as an individual fate, the financial and social burdens of which had to be borne by those afflicted and their families. To gain access to the help of doctors and nurses they either had to use their own resources or hope for the benevolent help of others. Illness was associated with poverty, a state of affairs which has still not been overcome in most countries on earth.

In the last 125 years systems for caring for the sick have developed in the Western industrialized nations, the economic, legal and social implications of which have gained enormously in significance in the course of time. Initially the medical care of industrial workers, who were organizing themselves, stood in the foreground: their labour was urgently needed during the Industrial Revolution and their efforts to share in political power were to be satisfied in this way.[1] If the perception of social responsibility so far lay with the charitable institutions, from the middle of the nineteenth century the state increasingly took on this task. The modern welfare state developed from that. Laws were created to regulate access to, and the financing of, the care of the sick. A comprehensive social legislation replaced what were previously purely professional regulations. Germany, which played a leading role in this development, established its legal, social and health insurance.[2] A new situation in the care of the sick came into being.

The socialization of illness

The socialization of illness is the decisive achievement of the modern welfare state. The circle of illness and poverty has finally been broken. People have access to medical care regardless of their social and economic status. Here there are important differences between the Western states. Thus for example in America there is a state system of basic care, financed by taxation, only for the poor and old (Medicaid and Medicare). The health system is primarily financed by private health insurance; 14% of the population have no insurance (in the Spanish-speaking population group the percentage is as high as 32%).[3] The level of individual care drops in ratio to income. In other states there are systems of universal care financed by taxation (e.g. the National Health Service in Great Britain), by social insurance (Germany), or by a combination of the two systems. The idea of the socialization of illness has been implemented most strongly in Germany. It finds expression in the so-called principle of solidarity, which prescribes compensation in solidarity for damage, risk, old age, income and family burdens.

However, despite fundamental differences, two things are common to all these systems: first a high degree of regulation and secondly a constantly growing financial need. Because of the constant development of the health-care systems and the tremendously rapid progress in medicine the legislators find themselves confronted above all with the following problems: the regulation of access to the health system, the determination of the extent of what it can provide, and the admission and control of providers and insurers.

Whereas there is a controversy in the USA as to whether a state welfare system for the whole population which is still to be created could be financed and would be justifiable,[4] in Great Britain and Germany the debate is on whether the existing systems can continue to be financed at the present level. With advancing medical possibilities and the demographic changes bound up with them, expenses are rising faster than new sources of income can be discovered. Since in the Western industrialized states the expenses of the health sector make up a considerable part of the Gross National Product – ranging from 8% in Great Britain through 9% in Germany to 14% in the USA – sickness is becoming a cost-factor in the national economy. There is talk of a cost-explosion, but this term is imprecise; there is largely an explosion of services on the one hand and a relative decline in income on the other. The Western states are in this dilemma. Thus there is a debate over the aims of health policy in which the key words are rationing, new models of taxation, liberalization of the market and prioritization. Here attention is being directed (too) strongly to the economic (and following that to the legal) aspects. No attention is being paid to social and political perspectives, though they would need to be at the forefront of a social discussion. So here once again we have the progressive economization of society.[5]

Healing as reintegration

In Germany, for example, this progressive economization is gradually upsetting the above-mentioned principle of solidarity. In Great Britain it is leading to further rationing in the NHS. In the USA the gulf in care between rich and poor is increasing. However, before offering criticism of economization it seems more meaningful first of all to define more closely some goals of health policy which are often concealed by economic goals.

It does not make much sense here to start with the WHO definition of health as a state of complete physical, mental and social well-being and not just the absence of illness and injury.[6] This description is too utopian. It is more useful to develop a concept of illness from the goals of health policy.[7] Instead of an ideal state of health for the individual (or society?), a reinforcement of the capacities of individuals and society to deal with illness could be a goal worth striving for. Here illness is to be understood as a concept with many levels; these are expressed better in English than in German, which has only one term. In English it is possible to talk of 'disease' as illness in the narrower diagnostic sense of symptoms and syndromes; 'illness' or 'sickness' as both a personal and a social phenomenon; 'mental disorders' in the case of psychological afflictions. So illness understood properly is not just a challenge for medicine, but for society. A precise and strong formulation of the concept of illness performs two important functions: as a diagnostic term it makes it possible to define precisely what services systems of medical care have an obligation to provide (and also to distinguish them from other systems of care in the welfare state); and as a term for a phenomenon which is both personal and social, it is opposed to a privatization of illness.

Similarly, healing must be understood as a social and not just as an individual event. Illness, above all severe and chronic illness, often leads to the withdrawal of the person concerned from society. These people withdraw themselves, but those around them also distance themselves from them. Thus in addition to the physical and psychological suffering there is a social isolation which is usually felt to be even more burdensome. Approaches to reform in medical care draw conclusions from this: they require care to be as local and as ambulant as possible. The world in which the patient lives is included in the planning for care. So-called house-physician models provide for active doctors becoming long-term supports for their patients in basic medical care; these doctors know their patients' worlds well and can be involved in the healing process. Thus participation becomes a goal of efforts at health policies: responsible patients and their families or close friends consult together with doctors and politics about how a health system is to be shaped.[8] It is here that the social dimension of healing comes in; here healing is shown to be reintegration into society. This becomes particularly clear in the care of the seriously or chronically ill. The social integration of e.g. chronic psychological patients can be regarded as an indication of the quality of a system of care.[9] As surveys in Sweden and Australia show, the population itself attaches priority to care of the most seriously ill over and above all economic considerations.[10]

Back to the privatization of illness?

However, in the face of the ever-growing tasks in the health sector, economic considerations stand in the forefront of public debates. There is no dispute that the financial situation of the health systems is under tremendous pressure. Yet it seems to me from the perspective of a health policy to be inadvisable to seek solutions exclusively in the economic sphere, as this will advance the fatal economization of medicine and society.

What solutions does the economy propose?

On the income side the possibilities seem to be largely exhausted. No one can increase tax quotas further. Rather, almost everywhere a lowering of tax quotas is sought. There is discussion in Germany as to whether the circle of contributors to legal sickness insurance should not be extended by raising the level of assessments[11] for contributions. The private systems of health assurance are energetically opposed to this particular proposal because they are afraid from their customers. We cannot hope for solutions here.

By contrast, a number of proposed solutions are being considered on the expenditure side. Here two levels are to be distinguished in principle: solutions at the level of the national economy (macro-) and solutions at the specific economy (micro-) level.

At the macro-level mention should be made first of a restrictions by the state on the level of expenditure. In Germany new legal regulations have been enacted within the framework of a so-called 'health' reform which fix both the levels of contribution by compulsory insurance and the budgets of doctors and hospitals.[12] As is evidenced by the British NHS, such measures lead to rationing.

A second measure is the liberalization of the health sector. That means on the one hand that the state withdraws from taxing the sector, and on the other that increased elements of competition are introduced in the sector, which is now understood as a 'market'. However, it may be doubted whether such a measure has a positive effect. The USA, which has largely liberalized its health sector, pays by far the most for it, namely around 14% of the GNP. Moreover, with 23%, the USA has the highest administrative costs. In Great Britain with its cost-effective NHS (around 8% of the GNP), after the introduction of supervised competition in 1991 the administrative costs doubled to between 11% and 16% of the NHS budget. In Germany they are running at 13%. The fear that more competition will merely drive up the costs of administration and advertising is thus justified and is confirmed in the case of German private health insurance.

Whereas a tax-financed system like the NHS is cost-effective from a macro-economic perspective, but keeps tending towards rationing, there are some weaknesses in the US system, which is predominantly organized in private economic terms. First, it is not in a position to be cost-effective at the macro-economic level; secondly, it tends to be selective in terms of risks or income and thus, thirdly, leads to a marked difference in care between rich and poor.

Finally, at the micro-level, illness or health is understood as something that has to be managed. Thus an economized concept of illness or health is introduced which leaves out the dimensions of illness mentioned above in favour of a partial aspect. Managed care systems, which are widespread in the USA and are being called for in Germany, are meant to give guidance on the one hand to those providing services (doctors, hospitals, etc.) and on the other to the (healthy) insured and to (sick) patients.[13] Here, in connection with the service providers, it is worth noting that around 80% of the volume of expenditure is determined by the decisions of doctors. By contrast, those who receive the services are, very much in market terms, customers: they can make a sovereign choice from the insurance offered them in accord with their wishes. They are to decide for or against particular services in the case of illness before this happens. The individual is to make private provision for risks, compulsorily assessed by income and resources. In the USA the result is that risks and income are factors in selection. The free choice of the 'customer' patient is praised as a reinforcement of self-determination.

This argument can also be heard in the German debate. However, here there seems to be some confusion between the 'sovereignty of the customer' and the participation of the person concerned.

First, no account is taken of the fact that health is a special commodity. In the economic theory of commodities it is called a 'public commodity' (i.e. it fulfils the criteria of being outside exclusiveness, competition and sharing). Secondly, in the health sector there is no real market: first, no one chooses the illness, and secondly there is a great asymmetry of information between doctor and patient.

All these proposed solutions have dangers, especially for the German welfare system, namely that the great achievement of the modern welfare state, the socialization of illness (and other social risks), will be sacrificed to the idea of the market. A privatization of illness of the kind called for in many Western industrial countries would close the old cycle which seemed to have been broken. Illness would again be connected with poverty.

Translated by John Bowden

Notes

1. Bismarck's 'Socialist Law' (1878) was the 'stick' and his social legislation (1883–9) the 'carrot' for the workers.
2. Compulsory insurance against illness (1883), industrial accidents (1884) and infirmity and old age (1889).
3. This and the following information on the health systems come from OECD Health Data, *Comparative Analysis of Health Systems*, Paris 1995.
4. As one contribution among many see R. Dworkin, 'Will Clinton's Plan be Fair?', *New York Review of Books*, 13 January 1994, 20–5.
5. Economization means the uncritical adoption of economic imperatives in other contexts of action. This does not mean a dichotomy between economic and social contexts but the dominance of the economic.
6. See the Constitution of the World Health Organization 1948.
7. This is also argued by a Swedish parliamentary commission, see Swedish Parliamentary Priorities Commission, *Priorities in Health Care – Ethics, Economy, Implementation*, Swedish Government Official Reports 5, Stockholm 1995.
8. In the US state of Oregon, but also in the Netherlands and Sweden, where this has been taken up, the population has been intensively involved in discussions on reforms of the health system. Despite all the legitimate criticism of the Oregon Plan, this participation is to be judged positively.
9. This view is put forward e.g. by W. Rössler, *Die psychiatrische Versorgung chronisch psychisch Kranker – Daten, Fakten, Analysen*, Schriftenreihe des Bundesministeriums für Gesundheit 77, Baden-Baden 1996.
10. Swedish Parliamentary Priorities Commission (n. 7); E. Nord, J. Richardson,

A. Street, H. Kuhse and P. Singer, 'Who Cares about Costs? Does Economic Analysis Impose or Reflect Social Values?', *Health Policy* 34, 1995, 79–94.

11. 'Levels of assessment' means the income level to which one is insured in the legal compulsory system.

12. Budgeting in this form was first introduced with the reform laws.

13. For managed care see e.g. M. Arnold, K. W. Lauterbach and K-J. Preuss (eds.), *Managed Care – Ursachen, Principien, Formen und Effekte*, Stuttgart and New York 1997.

Part II

Religion, Misfortune and Illness in the Pre-Industrial West

Jean Delumeau

To understand how attempts were made to cure illnesses and to cope with misfortunes in the pre-industrial West we need to undergo a real intellectual conversion and enter a universe which is no longer our own. I shall attempt to achieve this by presenting a certain number of documents at first hand. Some may prove astonishing.

Père Michel Le Nobletz, who preached in lower Brittany from 1610 on, discovered there 'disorders and "superstitions" which brought tears to his eyes':

> There were a large number of women who carefully swept the chapel nearest to their village. When they had gathered the dust, they threw it up into the air so as to have a favourable wind for the return of their husbands or children who were at sea. There were others who took the images of the saints in the same chapels and threatened them with all kinds of ill treatment if they did not bring about the prompt and happy return of those who were dear to them; and indeed they carried out their threats, whipping these images or putting them in the water when they did not obtain from them all that they asked for . . . One saw many who took great care to pour away all the water in a house when someone had died, for fear that the soul of the dead person might drown in it, and who put stones by the fire which each family was accustomed to light on the eve of St John the Baptist's day, so that their fathers and their ancestors would come and warm themselves there . . . In these same places it was an accepted custom to kneel before the new moon and to say the Lord's Prayer in its honour; it was also a custom on the first day of the year to make a place of sacrifice at the public fountains, everyone offering a piece of bread and butter to

the fountain in his village. Elsewhere on the same day they offered to these fountains as many pieces of bread as there were members of their families, judging who were going to die during the year by the way in which they saw the pieces thrown in their names floating on the water. But the offerings which many people made to the evil spirit were even more abominable. These poor people, thinking like the Manichaeans that there are two principles of good things and evil things, believed that the devil had produced the black grain or buckwheat; so after harvesting this last sort of wheat, on which the poorest of some provinces of the kingdom fed, they threw several fistfuls into the ditches surrounding the fields where they had gathered them to give a present to the one to whom they thought that they had the obligation.

Given this failure to understand Christianity, the vast majority of Europeans, above all in the countryside but also to a certain degree in the city, inevitably combined a whole series of beliefs and magical practices which came from an extremely distant past with the official religion, which was most frequently accepted without question. Since the historians and ethnologists of the European past have begun to occupy themselves with this question they have dug up a mass of facts that our humanist and bookish culture had for a long time refused to see, but of which the Protestant Reformers and their Catholic counterparts were well aware. In his *Dialogue concerning Heresies* (1529), Thomas More puts the following story in the mouth of his 'messenger'.

I can assure you that what I am going to tell you I saw with my own eyes. At Saint-Valéry, here in Picardy, there was an abbey in which St Valéry was a monk. Some hundreds of paces below it, in a wood, is a chapel where this saint is invoked especially against the malady of the stone: people come there not only from round about but also from England. Now there was a young gentleman who had married the daughter of a merchant. Having a little money to squander, which seemed to him to be burning a hole in his purse, during the first year of his marriage he took his wife on a journey abroad, with no aim other than to see Flanders and France, and to devote the summer to making an expedition in these lands. On the way, one of his companions started to tell him many strange things about this pilgrimage, so he decided to go somewhat out of his way to see if it was true, or to mock his man if he found it to be false – it was in fact this latter conclusion that he thought he would have to draw. But when they arrived at the chapel, they perceived that it was all true; and with their own eyes they found even more follies than the companion had related. For if in the other places of pilgrimage one saw wax legs, or arms, or other parts of the body hung up, in this chapel all the *ex voto* objects attached to the wall consisted of the sexual parts of men and women made from wax. As well as these objects, at the end of the altar there were two silver rings, one much larger than the other, in which each man placed his member: not in both, but some in one and some in another, for the two rings were not of the same dimension; one was larger than the other. There was also a monk, standing at the altar, who blessed Venetian gold threads. He distributed them to the pilgrims, telling them how they themselves or their friends were to use these threads against the stone: they were to tie them around their member and say I don't know how many prayers . . . Our gentleman had a servant who was a married man but a cheerful character: thanking the monk for the thread, he asked the monk to show him how to knot it around the sexual member of his wife. Since the monk was not a specialist in the art of tying knots, this seemed to him to be difficult since her sexual member was quite small. I need not tell you that everyone laughed, except the monk, who threw his rings and his threads in the air in a great rage and went off. It is not that . . . But listen. Good God, I had almost forgotten a detail which must not be omitted at any price. When this gentleman was on his knees in the chapel he saw a good woman of mature age approaching. She indicated to him the existence of a rite special to this pilgrimage, and more sure against the stone: she did not know whether he had been informed of it. If he submitted to it she was ready to wager her life that he would never have the stone for the whole of his lifetime. This is what he related: she took the length of his sexual member as the measure of a wax candle which would be burned in the chapel while certain prayers were related. This was the absolute remedy against the stone. When he had heard this – as a man who had a great fear of the stone – he went to ask the advice of his wife, but as a faithful Christian she did not like such superstitions. She could tolerate the rest quite well but when she heard mention of burning the candle she raised her eyebrows and, crossing herself, earnestly remarked, 'Good God, be careful what you are doing. Burning,' she said, 'is not pleasing to God. It will harm your sexual member, on my life; I beg you, beware of this sorcery.'

Abbé Germain Le Marc'hadour, who drew my attention to this text, points out that the 'messenger' in Thomas More's *Dialogue* is 'a young anticlerical tempted by Lutheranism' and 'hostile to the cult of saints and to pilgrimages, in which he lists various aberrations'. Thomas More is not in fact accepting his account as it stands, but he wants to show that if the Catholic Church does not sweep its own doorstep clean, it will become the sport of Protestantism.

In a remarkable work, *Religion and the Decline of Magic*, Keith Thomas has presented an extraordinarily rich picture of popular belief and behaviour in England on the eve of the Reformation. The English medieval church, he says – though this applies to the whole of Christianity – was a 'vast reservoir of magical power'. By offering a peck of oats to St Wilgerforte, a wife discontented with her husband could hope to get rid of him. People carried on their person *agnus dei*s (little wax loaves with the image of the paschal lamb on them), perhaps out of devotion, but also as protection against lightning and fire, to avoid drowning or death while giving birth. Other talismen were the rosary, and a fragment of the Gospel of St John as protection against storms, fever and evil spirits. In North Wales in 1589 people made the sign of the cross when closing their windows, leaving their livestock or going out of the house in the morning. And if misfortune struck someone or his animals, he was told, 'You didn't make the sign of the cross today,' or 'You didn't make the sign of the cross on your cattle.' When there was a storm, the bells of the village church were rung, since as everywhere else in Europe people thought that they would drive away thunder, lightning and evil spirits.

The sacraments too were drawn into the magic circle of a religion of the land and it was said that the mass acted 'as a charm on a viper'. The communicant did not swallow the host but took it away, thinking that with it he had an extraordinary force under his control: it could cure him if he was sick, and he was protected against misfortune. If he spread the host on his garden in the form of powder the caterpillars would be destroyed. Hence the instructions in the first Prayer Book of Edward VI that priests were to put the host in the mouth of the faithful. A criminal who took communion could imagine that he would escape punishment. Baptism did not just open up access to grace; it seemed necessary if the child was to live. It was said that some blind babies began to see when they were baptized. The head-dress of the new-born child was also baptized and it became a kind of talisman. Because of the popular meaning sometimes given to this sacrament, people would baptize dogs, horses and sheep. That a magical power was also attached to confirmation is proved by the fact that Elizabeth I was confirmed three days after she was born. According to Keith Thomas, Christianity and magic were thus inextricably mixed. Another proof is the widespread belief in fifteenth-century England that one could avoid sudden death by fasting all the year on the day of the week corresponding to the day on which the Feast of the Annunciation fell.

For us these facts relate to the mental structures of the pre-industrial age. It was very difficult, and sometimes impossible, not to try to affect natural phenomena by means of recipes which today seem to us to have no connection with the laws of nature. Hence the observation of P. Joutard about the Reformed regions of the Cévennes after quite a recent survey: 'Magical beliefs seem to be as varied in Protestant countries as in Catholic countries, being about anything from fantastic beings of a more or less diabolical kind to phenomena of the "evil eye" and spells.' Why, the sociologist R. Luneau then asks, should the revealed religions and rural traditions be irreconcilable? In the spirit of many black people, this African specialist notes that there is no discord between Christian faith and fetishist practice. For them, several sacred actions are better than one, and a spontaneous concordism allows them to reconcile what might seem irreconcilable to our Cartesian spirits.

Luneau has compared the image which African Christians still often have of the priest today with the image which French peasants until very recently had long held. The comparison is illuminating. In both cases the priests stands out as the healer, the seer, the magician, the one who knows the hidden things, conjures up the spirits of the dead and robs them of their power. He carries the eucharist to put out fires or to divert storms. He is a mediator between the population and the mysterious forces which threaten the collectivity. He is a being who gives security in a society in the grip of insecurity. Moreover, since human groups do not succeed in dominating in the long term the phenomena which make them insecure, the strictly scientific causes of which escape them because of their cultural level, every external religious contribution is necessary reinterpreted in terms of a magical model.

However, we can note historically that the two religious reforms in the sixteenth century, while rival, both tried to fight against 'superstitions' and in some way set priests (or pastors) against magicians. The latter became the object of growing suspicion on the part of the theologians and the judges. This has been brought out well in Lorraine from the end of the sixteenth and the beginning of the seventeenth centuries. As Nicholas Rémy wrote:

'All Christians are agreed in professing that the presence of sooth-sayers in the church is intolerable and the preachers damn them and curse them every Sunday.' Judges in Lorraine declared to some who had been warned that 'this kind of soothsaying does not come from any other source than the malign spirit', and that 'all these superstitions were true sorcery, forged in the devil's den'. When someone accused had tried to heal a bull by tracing signs of the cross on him with the left hand, and another (from Saint-Dié) had practised therapeutic absolutions with water drawn 'by night . . . from the river', their 'recipes' were thought to have been taught, not by 'a mortal person', but by a malign spirit', since only Satan, who 'hates nothing so much as the light and is called the prince of darkness', could have suggested recourse to such a medication.

On the other hand, notably in the seventeenth century, the church was particularly vigilant about the multiple manifestations of superstition prompted by the cycle of St John the Baptist. In several dioceses they were absolutely forbidden as tainted with 'superstition'. In others, attempts were made to channel the popular tendencies by Christianizing them. The *Catechism of Meaux*, from the time of Bossuet, is revealing in this respect:

Q: Why does the church show so much joy at the birth of St John the Baptist?
A: It does that only to perpetuate the joy that the angel had predicted . . .
Q: Is that why they light bonfires?
A: Yes, that is why.
Q: Does the church take part in these bonfires?
A: Yes, since in several dioceses, and particularly in this one, several parishes light a fire which they call ecclesiastical.
Q: What reason do they have to light this fire in an ecclesiastical way?
A: To banish the superstitions practised at St John the Baptist's fire.
Q: What are these superstitions?
A: Dancing round the fire, playing, holding festival, singing dishonest songs, throwing herbs on the fire, picking them before noon or when fasting, carrying them around, preserving them through the year, keeping brands or charcoal and other such things.

Bossuet's attitude to the tricky question of the St John the Baptist's fires seems to have been the most widespread one among the clergy of France, as is attested by a popular instruction of 1665 on the origin and manner of making the fire of the Nativity of St John the Baptist to remove the abuses and superstitions from it. As in a catechism, questions and answers alternate:

Q: What are the abuses which have been introduced into this

ceremony over the course of time?

A: Superstitions like making certain turns or circles round the fire and making animals do the same thing, and taking away little brands, coals, cinders, wearing girdles of herbs, throwing bundles of herbs and passing them over the fire . . .

Q: And with regard to the material of this ceremony, what preparation or decoration do they make?

A: In the middle (of the square) they set up a little stake of eight or nine faggots, but not using large pieces of wood, so that this fire does not last longer than the prayers that they chant and so that there are no bits of burnt wood that can be taken away to serve as superstitions . . .

Q: What is the order of the ceremony . . .?

A: While the fire burns, a lay officer pokes the wood to make it flare up and burn more quickly, and a clergyman of note remains by the fire to keep the people at their duties and prevent anyone from picking up and taking away wood or carbon so small that it could be used for superstitions and any other disorder. Finally, when everything is finished, some water is thrown to put out the fire that remains; the cinders are brushed away and the square is made clean, the carpet and the picture of St John are shaken. All this is to be done by the person in charge of the fire.

The St John the Baptist fires were controlled, sanctified and if possible restricted in number – the *Instruction* of 1665 asked the lords not to allow 'any particular fire'. We can see the suspicion of paganism attached to this piece of folklore and the efforts made from the seventeenth century on to Christianize it. This is a particular – but revealing – case of the struggle undertaken at that time in many ways by religion against a tenacious 'superstitious' mentality.

Further illumination on this incessant fight is cast by a last fact, chosen from thousands. It has been pointed out by T.-J. Schmitt in his work on the diocese of Autun:

The inhabitants of Reclesne came to invoke during childbirth a cardboard Virgin in a chapel of their church. After some prayers and an offering, the belly of the statue was opened to reveal there a little baby Jesus; then it was closed again piously with the hope of a happy delivery. The priest, having been ordered not to tolerate this superstition any longer (1689), took the step of surrounding the belly of the Virgin with an iron band and assured the authorities, perhaps prematurely, that the devotion was no longer practised.

However, at a time when techniques and medicine most often had no weapons against dangers and illnesses, what other recourse than these could one have against them? That is why the various Christian confessions tried to meet popular demand in this respect and respond to it by remedies and rites controlled by the church authorities.

Here, for example, is the procession of horses which under the Ancien Régime took place annually at the abbey of Saint Eloi in Noyon:

Every year, on 25 June, the anniversary of the translation of the relics of Saint Eloi, according to the martyrology of Noyon, the pilgrimage of horses took place: sick or vicious horses for whom the intercession of the saint was to obtain healing or a change; good mounts which his blessing was to preserve from accidents or illnesses. A number of farmers and others went there on foot, leading their animals and praying devoutly all along the way. They attended a solemn mass, before which the procession of horses, led by hand, began, to the singing of the hymn of the pontiff confessors. The horses were led round the outside of the chapel, and as the person leading a horse passed in front of the open door of the sanctuary he would stop, face the altar, and bow in a deep genuflection. The procession stopped behind the choir, and the celebrant, assisted by the deacon and sub-deacon, proceeded to bless a certain amount of water in a small container. This blessed water was then taken away by the pilgrims, who used it to mix the horses' feed, especially that of sick horses. Those whose horses had been impossible to lead took care to furnish themselves with a fistful of hair from the tail of the sick horse and participated in the procession holding this offering in their hands: then they put it on the steps of the altar. The others also put hair or coins there.

Another significant example is that of exorcism against the advance of glaciers. The people of Chamonix, who in the seventeenth century found the glaciers advancing into the valley and destroying or threatening houses and crops, on several occasions begged the successive bishops of Annecy to come to exorcize the 'mountains of ice'. Here is a witness on the matter:

The inhabitants of a parish called Chamonix showed the trust they had in the blessing of their bishop in a singular way. Chamonix had large mountains covered with ice . . . (which) . . . constantly threaten neighbouring places with ruin; and whenever the bishop paid a visit to this area the people begged him to go and exorcize and bless these mountains of ice. About five years before the death of our bishop these people made a deputation to him to beg him to go and see them once more in the fear that they had, so that, since he was growing older day by day, his age would not deprive him of this happiness . . . They assured him that since his last visit the glaciers had withdrawn by more than eighty paces. The bishop, charmed by their faith, replied, 'Yes, my good friends, I will go, even when I have to have myself carried there . . .' He went there and did what they wanted. I have a testimony made on the oath of the most notable people of this region in which they swear that, since the blessing given by Jean d'Arenthon, these glaciers have withdrawn to such a degree that at present they are an eighth of a league from the place where they had been before the blessing and that they have ceased to inflict the ravages that they did previously.

Four times a year, on 25 April and the three days before the Ascension, the clergy and the faithful went in procession across the fields to beg the protection of heaven against the scourges of the climate. Moreover, prayers and special processions took place to ask for the end of the drought or the cessation of rain. Six processions of the reliquaries of St Geneviève and St Marcel took place in Paris during the eighteenth century, after being authorized by Parliament: four times to obtain rain (1603, 1611, 1615, 1694) and twice to make it stop (1625 and 1675). In many vine-growing areas – for example round Paris – the custom was to take the Blessed Sacrament into the vines to protect them from worms and insect pests. The use of exorcisms used to be general: they drove away evil and misfortune. G. Le Bras has counted 120 documents in the archives of Doubs from the years 1729 to 1762 containing requests to the archbishop for formulae for exorcizing insects and rats.

Our ancestors, defenceless in the face of threats which seem to us to be natural but which they did not identify as such, thus felt the pressing need to resort to the weapon of exorcism. The '(Roman) Ritual for the Diocese of Agen' of 1688 provides a good example of prayers for driving harmful animals from crops, asking for rain or fine weather, putting an end to plague or famine, and dissolving storms and tempests. In this last case the ceremony included an exorcism. The instructions for the ritual first of all specify that the parish priest or his curate should ring the bells, light candles on the altar, and put on a violet stole and a cape of the same colour. Clergy and faithful are to recite the litanies of the saints and go in procession around the church if the weather allows, otherwise inside it:

'On returning to the church door the priest, with the cross in his hands and turning towards the storm', is to say:

Lord Jesus Christ, who made the heaven, the earth, the sea, and all that is in them, who blessed the Jordan and willed to be baptized in it, who spread out your most holy hand and your most holy arms on the cross and who by them have sanctified the air, we beg of you the limitless abundance of your pity and goodness. Deign to dissolve and destroy these clouds which I see disturbing the air in front of me, behind me, above me, to the right and to the left, so that the impious and demonic power which manoeuvres them may fail and be put to flight . . .

Cloud, may God the Father encircle you, may God the Son encircle you, may God the Holy Spirit encircle you; may God the Father destroy you, may God the Son destroy you, may God the Holy Spirit destroy you; may God the Father stifle you, may God the Son stifle you, may God the Holy Spirit stifle you.

This last prayer was punctuated by nine signs of the cross and followed by the exorcism proper:

I, a sinner, priest and minister of Christ, though I am unworthy, by the authority and virtue of this same God our Lord Jesus Christ, the emperor (*imperator*) supreme, not relying on myself and basing myself on my own power, I order you, most unclean spirits which stir up these clouds and vapours, by the virtue of this same God and our Lord Jesus Christ, by his most holy incarnation, by his baptism, by his fasting, by his most holy cross and by his passion, by his holy resurrection, by his splendid ascension, by his fearful return for judgment, by the merits of Mary most pure and ever virgin, by those of St (the patron of the parish) and by those of all the saints: come forth from these clouds and spread them over forests and uncultivated places, so that they cannot do harm to men and women, to animals, to fruits, to herbs and to anything related to human needs. By the same Lord Jesus Christ who will come to judge the living and the dead, and the age by fire.

He orders you, demons who stir up these clouds, he of whom a voice which came out of the shining cloud declared, 'He is my Well-Beloved Son in whom I am well pleased', he who purified the air by stretching out his most holy body on the most holy cross orders you. He who by his death conquered and chained you, your prince, and death, and will deliver you to the flames of eternal gehenna, orders you. He who, escaping from hell, rose from the dead, orders you. He who after forty days, veiled in a cloud, ascended to heaven by his own power, orders you. He who will come to judge the living and the dead and this age by fire orders you.

In all the exorcisms and benedictions mentioned above, it was the sprinkling of water which signified and brought divine protection. Hence the need for the clergy and the faithful always to have holy water available, which could be used not only in the ordinary liturgies but in the case of pressing danger. In 819 Rabanus Maurus wrote in his *De Institutione clericorum*:

> We bless the salt and the water for different uses by the faithful: against visions conjured up by the enemy, for the health of cattle, to drive away illnesses . . . For no other element in the world purifies and vivifies all things like water since, baptized in Christ, it is by water that we are reborn to live again purified. Water flowed from the side of Christ with the blood to invite us to use it as the sacrament of all sanctification and all purification. And the mixing of the blessed salt with the water is done by the authority of God, who ordered Elisha to throw some of it in a spring to cleanse the waters of Jericho. Thus the nature of salt is close to that of water and joined with it: they belong to the same element, have the same office and the same meaning, for water cleanses dirt and salt drives away putrefaction; the water brings cleanness and the salt produces sincerity; the water signifies a potion of wisdom and the salt the taste of prudence . . .

This pedagogical text illuminates the whole use of the sacramentals in the Catholic Church. By virtue of examples or affirmations from scripture, they were reputed to act on both the soul and the body, bringing healing, cleansing or protection to one person or another. The ritual of Lausanne printed in 1500 contains 'an exorcism and a blessing of the water' which are quite revealing, despite the grammatical weaknesses which make them difficult to translate:

> Prayer. Secure, Lord, your saving remedy for this creature of salt and water so that, where it shall be spread, it will serve the health of the soul and the body and bring about the destruction of worms and caterpillars and all animals who harm the fruits of the earth. For ever and ever, etc.
>
>   . . . You, creature of salt and water, I adjure you by the living God, by the true God, by the holy God. I adjure you by the true God who ordered you to flow from the fountain of paradise. I adjure you by the

one whose power converted you into wine in Cana of Galilee, who walked with dry feet on the sea and who gave you the name Siloam. I adjure you by the one who, thanks to you, cured the leprosy of Naaman the Syrian and who, when the prophet Elijah had added salt to you, purified you with these words: 'Holy water, pure water, water which washes away all stain and removes sins.' I adjure you by the living God to show yourself pure and not to retain any phantom but to act as an exorcized spring and as salvation for all believers. Wherever you are spread – on the harvests, on the trees, on the farms and the houses, in the corners of the bedroom, on the fields, the vegetables and the beet, on the domestic and useful animals – and for every being and every thing which tastes you and knows your savour, may you serve as a defence against the worms, the caterpillars, the rats, the snakes and all the animals which devastate the fruits of the earth and as a remedy and protection for life and health. May the devil himself, the worms, the caterpillars and all the animals harmful to the fruits of the earth be removed and flee afar. May the distance which separates heaven and earth, light and darkness, the just and the unjust, sweet and bitter also be between the fruits of the earth and the unclean spirit, the caterpillars, the worms, the rats, the snakes and all harmful animals. Protect those who have tasted you and who have received your aspersion from all harm that affects men, women, place, herds and animals; by the word and virtue of our Lord Jesus Christ who lives and reigns with the Father and the Holy Spirit.

The length of this liturgy and the content of its prayers are extremely significant. They show in exemplary fashion what the shorter 'benedictions' often express only in a minor way: an uncontrollable need for protection which the Catholic Church met, in the present instance, with a large panoply of reassuring rites.

This collection of blessings, conjurations and exorcisms has led me to ask a question. What replaced these reassuring rites in Protestant countries? Or where they maintained in a more or less underground way?

An answer can be obtained from a small book published in 1925 by a Lutheran pastor making an investigation at this time in his own region – Magdeburg. He found 'blessings' in use which certainly did not have the approval of the religious authorities. Here are two of them:

1. Blessing of the house

Most holy Lord Jesus Christ, you who were crucified, I beg you, protect this house and all the souls who live in it, whom you have purchased by your blood. On the cross, Lord Jesus Christ, you sacrificed your spirit for love of us. Cover this house with the blessing of the Most High. May the Holy Trinity bless this house. God, Father, Son and Holy Spirit, fill all this house – men, women and cattle – with rich blessings. May the most high name of Jesus bless all the human beings who enter and leave this house and keep them henceforth from all misfortune: sickness, plague and other dangers. Jesus, protect this house from perils of fire and water, from war and other calamities, from the misfortune of dearth and terrible poverty. May the holy name of Jesus with the nine angelic guardians be blessed. May the four holy angels stay at the four corners of this house and be its guardians and defenders so that no misfortune strike it henceforth coming from sorcery, demonic phantoms and other harsh scourges. May the cross of Jesus Christ be the roof of this house. May the three beams (of this cross) be the bars of its door. May the crown of Jesus Christ be its buckler and may his five holy wounds serve as its lock and wall. In this way may this house and all around it be blessed. Most honoured king of heaven, protect with your benevolent wings the fruits of the field, the gardens and the trees against the return of any misfortune. May we live happily in good health and as Christians. Amen. May God help us, Father, Son and Holy Spirit, Amen.

2. Blessing of the fire

Be blessed, host of fire: do not seize more than you have taken. I order you, fire, on pain of punishment in the name of God the Father who has created us (+), in the name of the Son who has redeemed us (+), in the name of the Holy Spirit who has sanctified us (+). I command you, fire, by the power of God who makes and creates all things, to remain tranquil and not to go further, as Christ stood in the Jordan when the blessed man John baptized him. I tell you, fire, on pain of punishment, in the name of God the Father (+), of God the Son (+), and of God the Holy Spirit (+). I order you, fire, by the power of God, keep low your flame as Mary, more excellent than all women, kept her virginity chaste and pure. Thus fire, soothe your fury. I order you, fire, on pain of punishment, in the name of God the Father (+), of God the Son (+), and of God the Holy Spirit (+). May Jesus of Nazareth, king of the Jews, deliver us from this calamity of fire. May he bless the fire and its flames so that it causes no damage, that it remains peaceful and does not proceed further. Fire must be tamed if it is not to cause great damage on earth. Many people doubt whether it will ever be calm. Let each one heed this instruction and take account of it. My God and judge (to whom I pray ardently), may I be blessed by your bitter sufferings and by your death.' After that recite three Our Fathers, turn round, fill your hand with earth, and throw it on the fire. Immediately it will calm down and not burn further forward, provided that no strident cry is uttered. Moreover anyone who is inflicted with epilepsy must attach this letter to his person for eight days. In this way the illness will depart and not return . . .

Now an almost identical text for exorcizing fire can be found on a flysheet printed at Königsberg in 1715. This is proof of a long circulation in time and space. Furthermore in 1926, in the neighbouring countryside the Magdeburg pastor collected a total of ninety 'blessings' of the kind that I have just quoted, amazed that they were being used after four centuries of Protestantism.

So a study of the various expressions of the need for security in the pre-industrial West (and even in a contemporary period) calls on us to follow the destiny and the preservation of reassuring practices from the earlier period beyond the break of the Reformation. Moreover it raises a very large question: is one of the major functions of religion – of all religion – to provide reassurance? The (very official) hymns of the Lutheran church also look after this need for reassurance.

Here are some examples. First, a Lutheran hymn from the seventeenth century at the time of a great storm.

1. O God, how terrifying is your wrath,
when you tread the clouds with violence,
and your powerful voice of thunder
sounds with tremendous din.
We poor and simple children of men
recognize your great power.
We are in fear and trembling,
for the heaven is filled with lightning and thunder . . .

6. Do not let your lightning burn
what you have given us for food.
Keep the thunderbolts away from us.
Make our bodies clean and safe.
Be at our side in all distress,
you on whom all hope is set.
Protect us from a sudden and evil death,
may your help not abandon us.

7. Cover with your hand
our body, life, house, cattle and goods.
Maintain the fruits of the earth
and all that shares your gift
from hail and floods,
from fire and tempests.
Protect us, God,
we want to praise you.

Another interesting piece from this collection is the hymn which is
addressed by a woman giving birth (a Czech Protestant text from the
eighteenth century):

2. See me here exposed
to an extreme torture.
I suffer inside and out,
and know of no help.
But you, my Lord,
deign to have pity on me
and from your throne send me
your holy presence.

3. The pains have begun,
the forerunners of delivery,
all my pores open with fear
letting through the sweat.
I go hot and cold,
horror overcomes me.
My heart stops with fear,
the fear of dying takes hold of me . . .

5. Deign to strengthen me
in my great swoon.
Care for me faithfully,
now and always.
Open my belly
when my hour comes,
that the fruit of my entrails
may see the day healthy and safe.

An important conclusion emerges from these two hymns and other
similar collections: clearly faithful Protestants drove their respected
churches to pray to heaven for their very concrete earthly distresses. To
disincarnate a religion would have passed over them.

However, a time has come when Western men and women have turned less than before to religion to protect them from earthly dangers. From the eighteenth century a laicization of the feeling of security began, and then accelerated. One significant instance is that for a long time in Catholic countries the church bells were sounded to drive away storms. But in the eighteenth century Benjamin Franklin discovered electricity and invented the lightning conductor. Moreover it was seen that the clappers of the bells attracted lightning. In 1787 the Parliament of Paris banned the sounding of bells during storms in areas within its jurisdiction.

The relationship between religion and misfortune began to change decisively. But does that mean that religion does not have nor ever will have the major function of reassurance outside immediate or imminent dangers? I would want to endorse some words of Père de Lubac:

> It can be argued that religion – and first of all faith in God – is a system invented by nature to *reassure* people who without it would be laid low by trouble and fear in the face of the hostile Mystery.
>
> But there is also another way of reassuring oneself: that of the rationalist, the short-term optimist, who does not rise to the feeling of this mystery and who proudly declares that there is no point in knowing it.
>
> Which of the two is nearer to the truth?
>
> Faith in God reassures us. That is undeniable, and there is no point in being embarrassed about the fact, as if the most intelligent had never felt anxiety or the most noble had never wanted to be delivered from it. Religion reassures us, not to procure for us a paralysing illusion or a beatific satisfaction, but to allow us to act. It puts trust in people so that they may prove worthy of themselves, that they may not succumb to the formidable crisis in growing which is created when the conscience is aroused at the departure from animality. It reassures human beings, but in order to communicate disquiet to them.

I would add: creative disquiet.

Translated by John Bowden

Illness, Suffering and Death as Related to Ancestral Sin

Jean-Claude Larchet

The Fathers are unanimous in relating illness, suffering and death to ancestral sin. In their view,[1] the source of illnesses, infirmities, suffering, corruption and death, as of all the evils which now affect human nature, is to be sought solely in the personal will of the first human being, in the bad use which he made of his free judgment, in the sin which he committed in paradise.

Although God is the 'creator of all things visible and invisible', he cannot be considered as the author of illnesses, suffering and death. Faithful to the teaching of Genesis according to which God's creation was originally wholly good (cf. Gen. 1.31), the Fathers agreed in thinking that man himself, in the first state of his nature, his condition in paradise, knew no illness, infirmity, pain, corruption and that in consequence death itself was a stranger to him.

Several Fathers (Athanasius of Alexandria, Basil of Caesarea, Augustine, Maximus the Confessor, Gregory Palamas) spell out this conception, indicating that the incorruptibility of the first man were due solely to divine grace.

However, they also note that since man was created free, it depended on his will whether or not he kept this grace, and thus remained in this incorruptibility and immortality which it bestowed on him, or whether he lost it. So in order to appropriate these qualities definitively, man had to remain united to God, with the help of the commandment which had been given to him for this purpose (cf. Gen. 2.16–17).

By choosing to follow the suggestion of the Evil One and to become 'as gods' (Gen. 3.5), i.e. gods outside God, Adam and Eve deprived themselves of this grace and from then on lost the qualities that they owed to it; by separating themselves from the Good they opened up human nature to all the evils. Because through Adam's fault human nature ceased to be conformed to God and to participate in his impassibility, his incorruptibility and his immortality, the whole of it 'fell sick with corruption'.[2] Athanasius of Alexandria and Gregory of Nyssa note that, losing the exceptional condition which it had originally through the presence of grace in it, it fell into an inferior condition. Gregory of Nyssa, Maximus the Confessor and John of Damascus affirm that while in the original mode of his existence man resembled the condition of angels, the condition of the new man resembled that of animals: his body acquired a material character, a density and an opaqueness that it did not originally have; it entered the current of animal life and the life of the senses, and from then on underwent the movements, the instability and the divisions which other beings of nature know. This new condition of existence is signified in Genesis by the coats of skin (Gen. 3.21) which, according to Gregory of Nyssa, symbolize man's material, animal character; the death which he hands down; and the fact that it is added to true human nature.

As archetype, principle and root of human nature of which initially he alone is the representative and which in principle in some sense he contains entirely, Adam necessarily hands down to all his descendants the evils which affect his nature, and these evils are communicated from generation to generation, in an essentially biological way.

Maximus the Confessor and John of Damascus emphasize that through man, the 'very grave illness' which affected him reached the whole cosmos, since he had been established by God as the mediator between God and the world. Instituted king of creation (cf. Gen. 1.28–30), he had power over all the beings that the earth contained, and his mission was to sum them up in him and to unite them with God, thus making them share in the order, harmony and peace from which his own nature benefited by its union with God, but also the incorruptibility and immortality received by grace. However, when Adam turned from God, nature ceased to be subject to him. Following his sin, disorder came about among the beings of creation, as it did with man. 'Cursed be the earth because of you' (Gen. 3.17), God says to the man, announcing the cosmic catastrophe brought about by his fault. From now on, according to Maximus the Confessor, the distinction and separation between beings became opposition and division. Since the human being had been deprived of the grace which had been his protection (cf. Gen. 3.7), and had lost his power of mastery over nature, he became weak in the face of it and subject to its attacks.

Evil spread all the more quickly and actively because since Adam had obeyed the devil, the devil could take power over man and usurp the privileges which God had granted him when he had made him master of the other creatures. In the domination of nature the 'prince of this world' replaced the 'king of creation'. Illness, the effect of Adam's fault, the consequence and form of evil which this engendered, was at the same time produced and reproduced, spread, developed, multiplied and reinforced. It sometimes even became incarnate, through the 'powers of darkness and misfortune', the devil and the demons, who then, as many of the Fathers stated, became one of the main sources of evil, showing themselves more often indirectly through them, but also sometimes directly, as in the case of possession.

Today this traditional conception is doubly problematical to some Christian theologians because of the gap between it and modern scientific theories. For the latter, on the one hand it is improbable (though this is still a matter of discussion) that humanity had a single founder and took its origin from a first man; on the other hand, illness, suffering, corruption and death have quite identifiable natural causes and seem inherent in life.

However, we may feel that the criticism of the traditional conception in the name of the facts of modern science confuses different points of view and indicates a failure to understand the perspective of the Fathers. It seems to me that, understood in its context and with its particular aims, this traditional interpretation need not be interpreted as a naive and pre-scientific theory; it can continue to be of interest without one having to understand it either literally or as unrealized symbolism.

First of all it has to be remembered that there were already numerous naturalistic explanations of illness in the patristic period and that some of them, characterized by a concern for rationality close to the modern scientific spirit (like those in the tradition of Hippocrates and Galen), were very widely adopted by Roman and Byzantine medicine, to the principles of which the Fathers largely subscribed without hesitation.[3]

Nevertheless, the Fathers found numerous advantages in referring correlatively to ancestral sin as the first explanation of illness, suffering and death.

1. Their position allowed them to be in agreement with Genesis 1, with Romans 5 and with various other remarks in the Old and New Testament. The rejection of the patristic conception implies the rejection of the almost unanimous interpretation of these passages of scripture by the Christian tradition down to our day and compels a reinterpretation of them in ways which are no longer satisfactory, whether because they

follow the fluctuation of scientific theories or because they consider that the sin of Adam signifies the actual sin of each individual.[4]

2. The main concern of the Fathers is to show that God is in no way the cause of the evils which affect his creation and has no responsibility for them.[5]

They exclude the fact that illness, suffering and death are inherent in material existence or life from the start. This idea was implied in different forms by the ancient philosophies (like Platonism and Neoplatonism), but also by different religious currents (Gnosticism, Manichaeanism, Origenism but also Pelagianism[6] – and a marginal Eastern current close to it, represented by Theodore of Mopsuestia, which appeared in reaction to Augustinianism). This idea seemed unacceptable to the Fathers, who thought it incompatible with the representation that one should have of God, since it signified either that the creation was the evil fruit of an evil, imperfect or degraded God, or that God was indifferent to his creation.

3. The conception which attributes the origin of evil to Adam's fault (and therefore will) breaks radically with the conceptions for which evil (and its effects) has an ontological cause and is one of the constitutive elements of the world (whether it is bound to an evil divine principle or is inherent in matter or life) and therefore seems natural and necessary, not to say eternal, and thus in some way normal, irremediable and definitive. It refuses to consider that evil is a fate or is trivial. It signifies that if evil had a beginning (in the will of the ancient Adam), it can also have an end (in the will of the new Adam). Contrary to fatalism and indifference, and thus to the passivity which derives from other religious or philosophical conceptions, it reminds people of their responsibility and implies a dynamic of struggle against evil and its different manifestations on both a physical[7] and a spiritual level.

4. Whereas according to St Augustine the guilt – and thus the responsibility – for original sin (conceived of as a sin of nature) is transmitted to the descendants of Adam, for the Eastern Fathers only the effects of ancestral sin have been transmitted: passibility (including suffering), corruptibility and mortality, along with a certain tendency to sin. So at birth not every human being shares responsibility for the evils which affect creation and will be responsible for and guilty of only the ills deriving from his or her own sins. Consequently the Eastern tradition is not led to envisage a direct link between the illness and suffering and the personal sin of the one who is affected by these. It notes that both the innocent and the holy can thus have to undergo serious illnesses and great sufferings, while sinners can live almost all their lives in good health and

shielded from suffering, a paradox which had already been emphasized many times by the Old Testament, and particularly strongly in the book of Job.

The modern conception which interprets the passages in Genesis about the sin of Adam as denoting the personal sin of each individual ends up by attributing guilt in a generalized way, and merely transfers to the personal level the collective responsibility which Augustinian theology (albeit less coherently) attributed to nature. If it is true that in some cases there is a link between the sin which each individual commits and the evils which can derive from individuals, those around them and their descendants, and if it is true that each individual by his or her own sins can contribute not only to the persistence of evil but also to its spread (which the Eastern Fathers readily recognize) both at the micro-level and the macro-level, evil has a nature and an extent in the universe which go beyond the power and scope of personal human wills.

5. The patristic conception can be criticized for making Adam a scapegoat who has to assume responsibility for all the evils in the world. However, in the eyes of the Fathers Adam's responsibility is mitigated by various considerations:

(a) The figure who really introduced evil into the world is the devil; by following his suggestion Adam merely opened the world to his power; and it is the Evil One who effectively extended evil throughout the universe, since from the moment that human beings were demeaned by their sin, they lost the dominion that they had over it;

(b) Adam was created in a childlike state; he was fragile and easily susceptible to the ruses of the Evil One;

(c) A rich patristic literature presents Adam as someone who repented immediately after his sin and obtained God's forgiveness; and in the traditional Eastern Christian icon of the descent into hell, Adam and Eve are represented as the first human beings to be saved by Christ;

(d) Adam's responsibility primarily relates to his own fault and the consequences which resulted from it for him; the consequences affecting his descendants relate to his position as a prototype of humanity and to the mode of engendering in which humanity finds itself as a result of his fault; from this perspective the transmission of his evil to his descendants becomes a fact of nature and does not derive from his personal will;

(e) Adam's guilt is shared by those who imitate him by sinning as he did (cf. Rom. 5.24) and who thus contribute to maintaining, not to mention spreading, evil in the world.

6. The patristic explanation does not claim to be a substitute for the naturalistic explanation of illness, suffering and death offered by

medicine; it does not present itself as a rival to scientific explanations. Science offers an explanation by physical causes; the Fathers offer a spiritual explanation which, while admitting that these physical causes are real (and while leaving science completely free to define them[8]), regards them as secondary to a first cause which is metaphysical. Far from excluding physical causality (whether biological, organic or functional), metaphysical or spiritual causality includes it and even considers it as necessary.

The interesting feature of the patristic conception is that it allows human beings to give a spiritual meaning to their illnesses and sufferings, and from the perspective of death to use them for their own spiritual edification; they are not just absurd phenomena, the effects of which are purely negative and destructive.[9]

7. The existence of the first human beings living in a state of relative perfection in which they escape sickness, suffering and death might seem incomprehensible and thus unacceptable, given our current knowledge of the laws of nature. That already caused difficulty for the people of antiquity, and Gregory of Nyssa thought it necessary to specify that 'the abnormal condition of the present conditions of human life are not enough to prove that human beings were never in possession of goods'[10] which are attributed to their original state. Gregory (and Maximus the Confessor has an analogous conception) considers that human nature originally had a different form of existence and thus obeyed different laws from those that we now know, to such a degree that we have become incapable of conceiving of others. The conception that the Fathers have of the origin of human beings corresponds to a different perspective from that of modern history and science, and for that reason should not be compared or contrasted with them. From a patristic perspective, the history of human beings as conceived of by human palaeontology is simply the history of a humanity which has departed from the conditions of paradise. The Fathers saw *homo habilis* as a representative of humanity, not as it emerged from the hands of God, but already deprived of its original state, at the lowest level of its 'involution' and beginning to develop in accordance with a new mode of existence. The original condition of human beings as presented by Scripture and the Fathers relates to a different temporality from that of historical knowledge: it does not belong to the time of sensible realities (*chronos*) but to the period of spiritual realities (*aion*), which escapes scientific history and relates to spiritual history. Without being atemporal (since it had a beginning in time and was called to experience a development over time, which moreover it inaugurated), the existence of Adam in his primitive state is

ante-historical, just as the human existence which follows the parousia will be post-historical. So spiritual history would not be 'outmoded' by historical science. The teaching of the patristic tradition about the origin of human beings is neither more nor less compatible with the actual facts of human palaeontology than the faith of the church in the eucharistic transformation of the bread and wine into the body and blood of Christ is incompatible with the facts of chemistry, or faith in the virgin birth of Christ and the resurrection of the dead is incompatible with the facts of biology and physiology, or again belief in the ascension of Christ is incompatible with the facts of physics and astronomy. In all these cases we have two different modes of apprehension, neither of which can be reduced to the other, their objects being different forms of being and becoming, the faith and spiritual knowledge corresponding to a domain where 'the laws of nature are transcended', a real supernatural mode of existence.

8. The patristic conception which relates illness and suffering to sin has the advantage of considering them in origin as evils that must be fought against. That helps to create a dynamic attitude for employing therapies and means for relieving suffering. I have shown elsewhere[11] how from the start Christianity, inspired by the attitude of Christ towards the sick, showed a concern to care for souls and bodies, and in order to do this not only proposed strictly spiritual therapies, but also had no difficulty in integrating the theoretical and practical contributions of secular medicine, even contributing largely to its development, while giving the therapy and healing a spiritual direction (referring them to God and making them symbols of salvation).

9. The conception of the Fathers coheres with the soteriological doctrine which they developed as a correlative.

Here, following St Paul, Christ is generally considered to be the new Adam, and the process of his saving economy is often presented in close relationship with the process of the fall of the old Adam, even corresponding point by point with it. This happens with Maximus the Confessor.[12]

Maximus the Confessor emphasizes that Christ, having been conceived without seed and engendered by a virgin, came into existence in a different fashion from other human beings, but one analogous to the genesis of Adam. By virtue of this, Christ did not have to undergo of necessity the effects of ancestral sin which all human beings had inherited by reason of their sexual engendering, but of his own free will assumed the passibility, corruptibility and mortality (but without the tendency to sin) which had affected Adam after his fall and then all his descendants.

For this reason, and by virtue of the power of his divinity which was united with his humanity in his person, Christ was able to deliver human nature from these evils and from the power which the evil powers had acquired over him through their intermediary.

Just as in principle Adam contained within him all the humanity which was to descend from him, so in the nature which he assumed Christ recapitulated all humanity, past, present and future (a Pauline theme which is developed particularly by Irenaeus of Lyons). Thus just as by its nature the effects of Adam's sin affect all human beings, so the effects of the saving economy of Christ, by virtue of the human nature which he has assumed, have benefitted all human beings, who will benefit effectively from it to the degree that they unite with him in the church which is his body.

Human nature, demeaned in Adam, thus finds itself restored to its original state by Christ and regains the privileges of the paradisal state. 'As in Adam human nature fell sick of corruption . . . so in Christ is has regained health,' notes Cyril of Alexandria.[13]

Christ has accomplished more than that, since he has not only saved but also deified human nature. But even when evoking this second aspect of the economy of the incarnate Word the Fathers do not lose sight of Adam, since they consider that Christ has brought to fulfilment the Creator's plan for the first man, a plan which had been diverted by his sin.

Moreover, Maximus the Confessor and John of Damascus emphasize that Christ fulfilled the mission of mediation between the creation and God which the Creator had entrusted to Adam, thus allowing all creatures to be united with humankind and God and to receive in their measure the benefits of the salvation and divinization accorded to human beings.

However, these benefits will be gained fully only at the end of time when 'all things become new'; human beings here on earth can only receive pledges of them.[14]

So while expecting that illness, suffering and death will be definitively abolished in the kingdom, they will have to continue to endure them. But through the grace of the saving economy of Christ these things have taken on another meaning: suffering has become a weapon against sin, and death has become the death of corruption and the destruction of death.[15] Though formerly fruits and instruments of sin,[16] and forms of condemnation of nature, if they are experienced or envisaged in Christ, they can become ways of salvation and means of attaining divine life and blessedness.

Translated by John Bowden

Notes

1. All the reflections which follow are developed, with references and quotations, in my *Théologie de la maladie*, Paris ²1994, 15–32.
2. Cyril of Alexandria, *In Rom.*, PG 74, 789B.
3. See my *Théologie de la maladie* (n. 1), 101–9.
4. See 3. below.
5. See, for example, Basil of Caesarea's treatise *God is Not the Author of Evil*.
6. It was with this heresy in view that canon 2 of the Council of Carthage (419) condemned the thesis that Adam was mortal by his nature and not his sin.
7. See 7. below.
8. See e.g. Gregory Palamas, *Triads*, II, 2, 30.
9. See my *Théologie de la maladie* (n. 1), 53–75; 'Du bon usage de la maladie selon les Pères', *Communio* 22, 1997, 17–28.
10. *Catechetical Discourses*, V, 8.
11. See *Théologie de la maladie* (n. 1), 77–132; *Thérapeutique des maladies mentales*, 43–132.
12. See especially *Quaestiones ad Thalassium* 21 and 61 and *Ambigua* 42.
13. See 2.
14. In my *Théologie de la maladie* (n. 1), 40–8, I have tried to explain why the physical effects of salvation, immediate in the human nature of Christ, are different for all other human beings.
15. This last point is emphasized by John Chrysostom, *Hom. in Matt.* XXXIV, 4. Maximus Confessor, *Quaestiones ad Thalassium*, 21 and 51, gives profound theological reasons for the change of meaning which suffering and death assume in Christ. See my article 'Ancestral Sin according to St Maximus the Confessor: A Bridge between the Eastern and Western Conceptions', *Sobornost/ECR*, 1998/1, and its development in chapter 2 of my book *Maximus le Confesseur, médiateur entre l'Orient et l'Occident*, Paris 1998.
16. Many evil passions and consequently sins were provoked not only by the attraction of pleasure but also by the tendency to flee pain and by the fear of death.

The Practice of Exorcism in the Church

Patrick Dondelinger

'*Exorcizare . . . est, per divina eum [spiritum immundum] adjurando expellere.*'[1] Augustine's classical definition of exorcism clearly indicates the aim and means of Christian exorcism: an unclean spirit (*spiritum immundum*), in other words a demon,[2] is driven out (*expellere*) by being adjured (*adjurando*) by the divine power (*per divina*). So the very existence of exorcism is based on a threefold belief: in the existence of demons, in the existence of a divinity stronger than the demons, and in the possibility that human beings can appeal to this divine power to drive away demons by addressing the spirits directly in the name of the divinity.

I. Exorcism among the first Christians

According to the Gospels, Jesus never practised any kind of exorcism: he drove away the demons by a simple word, pronounced on his own authority, without adjuration in the name of a divine power. It might be mentioned that in the Gospels adjuration in the name of God is what is done by diabolical powers: the demon which possessed a man (cf. Mark 5.7), the high priest in his accusation (cf. Matt. 26.63); in a paradox which is both tragic and comic they begin to adjure (*exhorkizo*) Jesus.

By contrast, Jesus' disciples subject the demons by adjuring them in the name of Jesus (cf. Luke 10.17). The first formula of Christian exorcism is reported to us in the Acts of the Apostles, when Paul drives out a spirit 'in the name of Jesus Christ' (cf. Acts 16.17).

If the way in which Jesus drove out demons is a unique feature in the history of religions, precisely because of the adjuration which constitutes exorcism, the practices of his disciples in this respect take up the classic scheme of the ritual adjuration of demons as it also appears in Judaism and in the other ancient cultures.[3]

Though we have to reconstruct the practice from texts which are far more apologetic than descriptive, the exorcisms of the first Christians have some distinctive features: sobriety, gratuitousness, a surplus of eschatological meaning which goes beyond the act itself and the person of the exorcists, and an efficacy which is all the more amazing since it contrasts with the poverty of the technical means used. According to the Christian authors of the period, this is what makes Christian exorcisms special, and they had to defend it against the competition from non-Christian exorcists and the accusations of occult magic which were directed at them by their Jewish and pagan detractors.

If the adjuration in the name of Jesus already intrinsically constitutes a profession of faith in his divinity, the therapeutic success of such an adjuration in a way constitutes the practical proof. Hence the importance of exorcism for the propagation of Christianity in a late antiquity which was particularly thirsty for salvation.

Apart from the great importance of the first centuries of Christianity for the history of the church, there can also be numerous parallels between this period and the current situation in non-Western cultures. Hence the interest in concentrating on the founding period of Christian exorcism.[4]

II. The discipline of exorcism in the early church

Very few, indeed virtually no, Fathers of the church fail to mention exorcism, putting it in the general view of the ancient world which saw demons at work everywhere.

In the first canonical regulations, those who have been exorcized appear as a specific category in the Christian community, for whom, if the case arose, special places, if not special adjacent buildings, were reserved in churches. Exorcistic therapy, which for the most part was practised by the community, combined prayers, incubations (a rite which involved spending the night in a sanctuary), fasts, liturgical gestures and adjurations.

We can note three main groups among those on whom Christian exorcism was practised in antiquity: the sick, those possessed and in a trance, and the catechumens. However, this distinction is somewhat artificial, deriving from a modern segmentary mentality, whereas the view of the world held by the first Christians was characterized precisely by its holism, combining in the same logic of adversity sickness, death, the demons, the devil, sin and pagans.

In keeping with the view of the ancient world which saw a close connection between illness and the demonic world, Christians were asked to exorcize the *sick*, a function which made them very useful, if not indispensable, to society. Here they seem to have combined prayers; exorcisms strictly speaking, in which the demon of sickness was adjured to depart; and medical-hygienic therapy.[5] We should note that there is nothing original in such a therapeutic combination; it corresponds to the medical practice of the time. If there was any Christian originality, it did not lie at the level of technique but at the level of the spirit in which it was performed: that of the love of God and love of neighbour.

I would describe the *possessed, strictly speaking*, as people regarded as inhabited by a demon which manifests itself through them at moments of violent crises, characterized by the trance of possession. The relative frequency of the possessed in antiquity can be explained by the general propensity of people at that time to give bodily expression to conflicts and individual and collective traumas; this was particularly prominent in an age of anxiety and profound upheaval. The vast majority of the possessed who were exorcized seem to have been Christians, but the writers also mention non-Christians. Some of the last converted are a cure by exorcism; others did not.

The attractiveness of Christian exorcism for these people can be explained by the fact that it allowed them to give expression to misfortunes escaping from the very depths of individuals and the group, while giving them a place through demonological language in the counter-logic which sees the victory of the Christian God and his visible and invisible champions. Through exorcism the psychodramatic expression of evil became possible and made sense, at the same time allowing the community to experience the liberating goodness of God, who triumphantly went out against the logics of hatred, dereliction and exclusion.[6]

Within the category of the possessed are also recent converts to Christianity who found themselves possessed by the gods of their own religion, most often after a transitory return to the practices of their ancestors.

During the course of the crisis of possession, these ancient gods surfaced as demon possessors; Christian exorcism freed those possessed by them, at the same time helping them to adhere fully, body and soul, to the new religion. In these circumstances exorcism took on an unrivalled apologetic dimension: in the grip of the Christian adjuration, the pagan gods had to confess that they were only wicked demons, before yielding to the orders of the Christian exorcizer and thus recognizing the goodness and superiority of the new God. And as described by the Christian authors of antiquity, the therapeutic function of exorcism became blurred, in favour of its apologetic function.

The third group of those on whom Christian exorcisms were practised was that of the *catechumens*. In Christian antiquity, initiation at baptism in fact included a number of exorcisms, culminating in a solemn final exorcism by the bishop. That marked the end of the scrutinies, which were concerned to examine closely whether the catechumen was from then on free from any hold of the devil which had been gained as a result of the cult of idols or the practice of vices. If baptismal exorcism, the only form for which we have any large quantity of documentation, is based on the exorcism of the possessed, it is partly because of a religious logic which lumps together paganism, sin and diabolical possession, and also because baptismal initiation, deliberately dramatized, in fact brought on real crises of possession in the case of certain catechumens. When applied to new-born babies, these same baptismal exorcisms served as an argument for the doctrine of original sin.[7]

The liturgical reforms following Vatican II proceeded to eliminate the adjurations driving out the devil as the customary preliminaries to baptism. While at least in the original Latin the new rituals of baptism keep the term 'exorcism', this is no longer exorcism in the technical sense of *adjurando per divina expellere*. Those responsible for the liturgical reform justified this change by a desire not to traumatize the faithful by dramatic adjurations; the fact is that the theologians themselves no longer thought of the person who had not been baptized as possessed by the devil.[8]

It seems that the early church also knew exorcisms of animals, objects and places alongside exorcisms intended for persons. We find such exorcisms in later rituals down to the Roman Ritual of 1952.[9] Here is a reflection of a demonistic view of the universe flavoured with a degree of Christian dualism: anyone who has not explicitly been exorcized is implicitly possessed; and the transition into the realm of the sacred requires a preliminary exorcistic purification.

III.The function of the exorcist

Exorcism, at first regarded as a charism, tended to become an institutionalized function, largely in order to avoid abuse, which became all the more tempting when prestige was attached to the performing of exorcisms.

For example Tertullian, in a piece of polemical apologetic contrasting the simple efficacy of Christian exorcisms with the knowledgeable and onerous pagan incantations, thinks that exorcism is within the power of any Christian,[10] while Origen, though accepting the existence of unworthy Christian exorcists, says that the people who exorcize are usually ordinary folk.[11] Origen presents this as an argument in favour of the power of Christian exorcism; however, to our eyes this passage is also an indication that at all times exorcism has been the prerogative mainly of popular circles, with their specific forms of religion.

From the end of the third century we can see a concern to put the function of the exorcist within the orders of the church, although exorcism essentially remains linked to charism: ordination is only in fact a recognition of this charism. However, as the function of the exorcist passes into the hands of the minor orders, and rapidly itself becomes a stage towards the priesthood, we can also see the ordination of people who do not have the charism but on whom ordination is to confer the faculty of exorcizing. From the fifth century on, the office of exorcist became purely formal, and was abolished by Paul VI in 1972, along with the other minor orders. In the Catholic Church, still from the perspective of the prevention of abuses, the practice of the exorcism of those possessed has thus long been reserved to priests who, in addition to having certain personal qualities, have received a special mandate from the local bishop.[12]

Now even before it was institutionalized, exorcism seems to have been reserved essentially for men: for Tertullian, the existence of a woman exorcist is already an indication of the heretical character of the group to which she belongs.[13]

IV.The later development of the practice of exorcism

At the end of late antiquity and in the Middle Ages, exorcism becomes the prerogative of the saints, present personally or in the form of relics. Healing takes place through a personal relationship between the possessed person and his or her God, established through the saint; he shows the liberating compassion of God and at the same time, if need be, settles social conflicts.

Furthermore, we should not forget the precarious living conditions and limited technical means in an agricultural civilization; hence the prime importance of exorcisms aimed at providing physical safeguards or healing for men and women, their food and their cattle; protecting against cosmic elements like storms and drought; and driving out rats, mice and other noxious pests.[14] Nor is it a coincidence that the abandonment by Vatican II of such exorcistic adjurations present up to the Roman Ritual of 1952 took place at a time in which the technical mastery of the universe by human beings led to an almost idyllic vision of the relationships between human beings and other creatures – as attested by the ritual of Benediction in 1984 – focussing the rites of the church merely on the mediation of a spiritual salvation, through the praise of God and sanctifying grace.

On the other hand, during the second half of the Middle Ages (thirteenth to fifteenth centuries), the exorcism of the possessed seemed to fade somewhat in the face of the practice of personal pity: inner conversion took over from the expulsion of an external devil.

This returns with the Renaissance, an age of anxiety and violence. Among other things, its internal tensions were manifested and externalized in the witch hunt, which was succeeded, through interiorization, by the massive appearance of cases of possession, in both Catholic and Protestant countries.

This period stamped the church's practice of exorcism in two ways: the normative codification of the rite of exorcism and the practice, pushed to the extreme, of banning its performance in public.[15]

In a concern to purify religious practices and to be open to secular sciences, Rome proceeded to produce a ritual of exorcism of the possessed which would apply to the whole of the Latin Church. This was the ritual of exorcism in the Romal Ritual of 1614, which remained almost identical until the last edition in 1952. In principle it is still in force in the Catholic Church of the Latin rite, although a new ritual of exorcism, confidential and interim, was sent to Conferences of Bishops in 1990.

If the formulae of exorcism in the Roman Ritual of 1614 merely take up schemes of adjuration from antiquity, the *praenotanda* introduce innovations, notably in recommending a distinction between illness and possession. This differential diagnosis is to be made through trial exorcisms which attempt to provoke the appearance of three empirical signs[16] thought to come directly from the devil, because they were otherwise inexplicable to the people of the time. This distinction between possession and illness, characteristic of the modern era but alien to the view of the ancient world and to contemporary epistemologies, seems to have been maintained down to the present day.[17]

The modern era has also experienced an extraordinary interest by the media in exorcism, which is both polemical and manipulative. Exorcisms have been performed publicly, sometimes in truly theatrical settings.[18] The therapeutic function of exorcism is completely set aside in favour of its apologetic power over against Protestants and others who are sceptical about supernatural Catholicism, not to mention the occasional denunciation of witches by the possessed. Exorcisms now produce such social and political tension that reasons of state have put an end to a practice thought to be both superstitious and a threat to public order.

In fact exorcism is becoming secularized, from the magnetism of the eighteenth century through the hypnotism of the nineteenth century to psychoanalysis and subsequent psychotherapies in the twentieth century.[19] If therapies have changed, it is because Western men and women have themselves changed. The expression of their ills has passed from a holistic somatization to a rational verbalization, which has largely been met by a scientific therapy that has taken over from the religious rite as an instrument of physical and psychological help.[20] When Western men and women, disappointed by the progress of scientific techniques, sometimes turn nostalgically to therapeutic rituals including exorcism, they sometimes forget that the efficacy of these rituals calls for a different worldview from that of the modern West, marked by the breaks introduced by scientific discoveries and Christian faith, with its distinction between physical and psychological health on the one hand and its theological and anthropological orientation on the other, an orientation which has resulted in a loss of both fear and interest in the world of demons.

V. Practices of exorcism in the contemporary West

In the West, the adjuration of demons is now becoming the prerogative, indeed the distinctive mark, of circles on the edge of society and the church. In keeping with the dynamic inherent in the sectarian practice of exorcism, it is no longer a factor in healing and social integration, as in traditional societies, but on the contrary leads to exclusion and imprisonment in pathology. Misunderstanding and the rejection that the adjuration of demons necessarily brings about in the church and in contemporary Western society then serves to magnify the controversial identity of the peripheral group. The original healing function of exorcism is perverted in favour of polemical attestation; in the face of subsequent inability of exorcism to produce a true cure, the absurd suffering brought about by the administration of the adjuration is reinterpreted as a sign of divine election and sacralized as a magical means of obtaining one's own salvation and that of others.

The pernicious perversion manifested by a large number of those who in the Western Catholic Church propagate the practice of the adjuration of the devil caused a sensation when a young student, Anneliese Michel, died during official exorcisms carried out by the Catholic Church.[21] This event, which took place in 1976, in Klingenberg, a small town in South Germany, also brought out the differences in sensibility which exist between one local church and another.

If the Klingenberg church has made it impossible for exorcists to function in the Germanic churches, feelings are very different in France,[22] where each diocese has its official exorcist who is sometimes listed as such in the telephone directory. The exorcists of the diocese of Rome witness to a practice which one can describe as 'baroque', taking up the demonological treatises of the seventeenth century.[23]

Even if the official exorcists of the church of France are submerged by requests for exorcisms, only a very tiny proportion of them practise the ritual adjuration of demons. However, this is prominent in circles of the charismatic renewal and among those who cultivate a traditional and popular piety which attaches great importance to religious marvels and rites of protection.

Polemic over exorcism within the church, engaged in by a militant minority which fears the abandonment of the old adjuration of the devil in favour of prayers which are more adapted to the representations of evil in Western culture and contemporary theology, seems for some reason to be delaying the reform of the ritual of exorcism, which remains one of the few rites for which no revised ritual in the spirit of Vatican II has yet been proposed.

This situation in itself already bears witness to how small a place the obtaining of psychological and social help through the religious rite occupies in the life of the contemporary Western Catholic Church. It thus calls attention to the primordial role of the cultural and ecclesiological context for the existence and efficacy of such practical therapeutic rituals. The rite of exorcism, which, in so far as it is sacramental, forms part of those rites which 'in accordance with bishops' pastoral decisions . . . can . . . respond to the needs, culture and special history of the Christian people of a particular region or time',[24] in fact raises in a particularly pressing way the question of the nature of Christian salvation and its effective realization for men and women in their everyday lives.

Translated by John Bowden

Notes

1. Augustine, *De beata vita* 3, 18, 12–13.
2. For the different names for demons cf. e.g. Patrick Dondelinger, 'Satan dans la Bible', in Frédéric Masquelier (ed.), *Encyclopédie des religions*, Paris 1997, II, 1463–7, supplemented by id., 'Quelques repères au sujet du diable et ses démons', *Prêtres diocésains*, February 1998.
3. Cf. Klaus Thraede, 'Exorcismus', *Reallexikon für Antike und Christentum* VII, 1969, 44–117; Dieter Trunk, *Der messianische Heiler. Eine redaktions- und religionsgeschichtliche Studie zu den Exorzismen im Matthäusevangelium*, Freiburg, Basel and Vienna 1994.
4. Cf. here Joseph Dölger, *Der Exorzismus im altchristlichen Taufritual. Eine religionsgeschichtliche Studie*, Paderborn 1909, to be supplemented by Ann Elizabeth Leeper, *Exorcism in Early Christianity*, doctoral thesis, Duke University 1991.
5. Cf. e.g. the classical study by Adolf Harnack, *Medizinisches aus der ältesten Kirchengeschichte*, Leipzig 1892.
6. Cf. Peter Brown, *The Cult of the Saints. Its Rise and Function in Latin Christianity*, Chicago and London 1981; id., *Society and the Holy in Late Antiquity*, Berkeley and Los Angeles 1982.
7. Cf. Dölger, *Exorcismus* (n. 4).
8. Cf. Balthasar Fischer, 'Baptismal Exorcism in the Catholic Baptismal Rites after Vatican II', *Studia Liturgica* 10, 1974, 48–55.
9. Cf. Elmar Bartsch, *Die Sachbeschwörungen in der römischen Liturgie. Eine liturgiegeschichtliche und liturgietheologische Studie*, Münster 1967.
10. Cf. Tertulllian, *Apologeticum* 23, 4.
11. Cf. Origen, *Contra Celsum*, 1, 6.
12. Cf. *Codex Iuris Canonici*, can. 11.72; Congregation for the Doctrine of the Faith, *Epistula Ordinariis locorum missa: in mentem normae vigentes de exorcismis revocantur, die 29 n.Septembris a.1985, Acta Apostolicae Sedis* 1985, 1169–70.
13. Cf. Tertullian, *De praescriptione haereticorum* 41, 6.
14. Cf. Adolph Franz, *Die kirchlichen Benediktionen im Mittelalter,* Freiburg 1909 (2 vols).
15. Cf. Patrick Dondelinger, 'Le rituel des exorcismes dans le Rituale Romanum de 1614', *La Maison-Dieu* 183/4, 1990, 99–121.
16. To speak or understand unknown languages; to reveal distant or hidden things; to show strength beyond one's age or natural condition.
17. Cf. *Catechism of the Catholic Church*, no. 1673.
18. Cf. e.g. the classic study by Michel de Certeau, *La possession de Loudun*, Paris 1970.
19. Cf. Henri F. Ellenberger, *The Discovery of the Unconscious. The History and Evolution of Dynamic Psychiatry*, New York 1970.

20. Cf. Antoine Vergote, 'Religion, pathologie, guérison', *Revue théologique de Louvain* 26, 1995, 3–30.

21. Cf. Johannes Mischo and Ulrich J. Niemann, 'Die Besessenheit der Anneliese Michel in interdisciplinären Sicht', *Zeitschrift für Parapsychologie und Grenzgebiete der Psychologie* 25, 1983, 129–93.

22. Cf. Isidore Froc (ed.), *Exorcistes*, Paris 1992.

23. Cf. Gabriel Amorth, *Un esorcista raconta*, Rome 1990.

24. *Catechism of the Catholic Church*, no. 1668.

The Healing Power of Faith. Outline of a Therapeutic Theology

Eugen Biser

The scheme

According to a much-discussed thesis, the future of the world will no longer be shaped by political or economic conflicts but by the 'clash of civilizations', to quote S. P. Huntington's term. That in itself already means that the religions of the world will be put in a hitherto unimagined situation of conflictual proximity. If this is not to lead to dangerous conflicts, initiatives towards mutual understanding are indispensable. This in turn requires that the standpoint of those concerned to achieve this understanding should be defined as exactly as possible. In the view of Romano Guardini there is the threat of a conflict above all between Christianity and Buddhism, since their founders each strove with the same mind, but towards different goals. Both Jesus and Buddha intervened in people's lives, one to raise them up to become children of God, the other to bring them low with the aim of diminishing suffering. Thus Buddhism proves to be the prototype of an ascetic religion focussed on taming passions and quenching the will to live. In defining the standpoint of Christianity it then has to be said that, unlike Buddhism, Christianity *is not an ascetic but a therapeutic religion.*

Whereas Buddha, faced with the oppression of human life and the self, promises the quenching of the passions and thus of the heart of all suffering that people cause one another, Jesus knows that he has been sent to heal the 'broken hearts' and to raise to people from their fallenness, in the twofold meaning of the expression: those who have been smitten with the wound of death.

The decisive proof for this thesis was provided by the discussion of the honorific titles of Jesus, which according to Ferdinand Hahn produced the result that the historical Jesus did not claim any of the titles attributed to him by the New Testament, so that he called himself neither Messiah nor Son of Man nor Son of God, but did allow titles with which he in fact introduced himself and with which he was also invoked in the early church in the prayer, 'Help, Christ, you are our sole physician.'[2] This is confirmed by his remark, 'Those who are well have no need of a physician, but those who are sick; I came not to call the righteous, but sinners' (Mark 2.17).

However, the saying needs explanation in two ways. In the first part of the sentence it is by no means a group of those in need of salvation to whom Jesus gives his help, distinct from those who, since they are 'well', do not need his help; rather, here Jesus is singling out from all those who in his eyes are sick the particularly difficult group of those who are unaware of their illness and therefore are doubly in need of his attention, because in their case not only their suffering but also a block in their consciousness needs to be overcome. As for the 'sinners' to whom Jesus knows that he has been sent, those gathered around his 'table of sinners' are not failures in the moral sense but those who are socially outcast and despised.[3] Jesus draws them particularly close to him, with the result that in the eyes of the establishment he seems to be a threat to the existing order of society; this is an occasion to cast him out and kill him 'outside the camp' (Heb. 13.13).

However, for the theological interpretation of this message this means that the therapeutic dimensions which are pushed into the background by the didactic character of the account must be rediscovered and again be given a place in theology. The outline of a therapeutic theology aimed at here is not a special form of theology like dialectical or political theology; rather, it is an attempt to bring theology back to its traditional – and truly appropriate – basic form and, in accordance with its basic task, to put it at the service of those who have been injured, people who are suffering in mind and body.

The question now, however, is whether faith can in fact heal. The answer given repeatedly in the Gospel, 'Your faith has made you whole', sounds no less fundamental. Thus in these earliest of phrases Jesus is by no means claiming for himself success in healing. Rather, he is attributing them to a faith which acts as an independent entity. This brings out most clearly that in fact he could heal.[4]

The diastasis

Leaving aside such obscure practices as 'praying for health' and 'spiritual healing', that sounds almost like a fairy-tale from a time long past. What has happened in the meantime is the history of a diastasis which already began in the New Testament period; it led to the collapse of the priestly image of the physician and finally to the complete transfer of the healing competence of Christianity to scientific medicine. That was not only reflected in the way in which theology presented itself but also had a decisive cause here. Theology was developed into a scientific system.

This development was imposed from within, but equally from the outside. From within, theology yielded to the need to interpret faith in an understandable way, because faith always needs to be understood from its centre – which is given with the divine revelation. The outside pressure was the need to offer justification against objections and attacks. The landmark of this development can be found already within the Gospel in the pericope of the healing of the paralysed man (Mark 2.1– 12), which was the focus of particular attention, as the history of early church art shows. Originally it was told as a moving story of faith, but in the final form in which it has been handed down it has been developed into an argument, so that by his miraculous actions Jesus seems to be justifying the forgiveness of sins which was practised by the primitive community but rejected by its Jewish neighbours.[5]

In this apologetic self-justification the philosophical categories were used only defensively. However, at an early stage, above all in Alexandrian theology, they were used constructively. Looking back, Augustine says that the theologians, recalling the silver and gold vessels 'borrowed' from the Jews at the exodus from Egypt, had taken over the thought-forms of Platonic and Aristotelian philosophy in order to present the message of the gospel in a 'scientific' form, i.e. one which could be introduced into scholarly discussion.

As time went on, however, the co-operation developed into confrontation, especially in the ambitious attempt to win back for Christian faith the territory in Spain lost to Islam. For here the missionaries came up against an Aristotelianism interpreted in Averroistic terms. They had nothing to set against its developed conceptuality until Thomas Aquinas in his *Summa contra gentiles* – aimed at the Spanish 'pagans' – gave them comprehensive help in argumentation.[6] In this confrontation the mutual dependence of theology on philosophy and vice versa remained undisputed. That changed when René Descartes cut the link between the two by detaching the cause of philosophy from the two pegs of tradition and authority and finally referred it to himself with the principle '*cogito ergo sum*'. Quite consistently, with Kant that led to doubt in the traditional definition of the relationship between the two. For in his work on the *Conflict of Faculties* the question arose whether philosophy, which was regarded as the handmaid of philosophy, was in fact following her mistress or whether she was not carrying the torch and thus taking over the key position.[7]

The reaction of the theologies divided by the split in faith was one of sheer panic. Whereas in despair Protestant theology threw itself into the arms of the Hegelian system, Catholic theology withdrew to the position of a *philosophia perennis* of a neo-scholastic type. Catholic theology had to pay for this retreat with a loss of contact with the present; Protestant theology discovered too late, as Karl Löwith showed in his acute analysis, that it had joined what was basically an atheistic system.[8]

If we reflect on this and accept with Horst Baier that in the meantime Plato and Aristotle have been driven from the field by Epicurus, the key witness for a post-modern, hedonistic mentality, the crisis of orientation to which present-day theology has fallen victim will become clear. And this is all the more a burden, since in the course of the de-Hellenization debate it has also become clear how little Hellenistic thought-forms, despite the apparent correspondence between the Logos of Heraclitus and that of John, corresponded to the gospel way of thinking.[9]

Lost dimensions

As theology became scientific, not only its therapeutic but also its aesthetic and social dimensions were lost. Jesus thought primarily in pictures. He was not only a figure in the history of religion and faith, but also a key figure in the history of language and the spirit. To communicate the notion of the kingdom of God which was central to his message, in the parables he created a sign world of his own made up of pictorial motifs. Over wide areas theological thought also followed this approach. The Platonic notion of ascending to the vision of the ideas remained a key factor for Gregory of Nyssa (the ascent of Moses), for Augustine in his vision in Ostia, and even for Bonaventura's *Itinerarium mentis in deum*, especially as at the same time Bonaventure orientated this work on the vision of the cross experienced by Francis of Assisi, the father of his order. With good reason, in Michelangelo's creation of Adam, with his left hand the Creator is grasping a group of putti-like figures: embodiments of the ideas in accordance with which, in this pictorial tradition, the creatures were sketched out and realized by God.

But then, at the height of the Middle Ages, the thesis became established that one cannot argue with images and that therefore no doctrines can be derived from images: *theologia symbolica non est argumentiva*. Thus there began an iconoclasm within theology which led to the systematic displacement of pictorial motifs by concepts. And with the images the aesthetic dimension was also completely rejected. But the gain turned into a disaster. For in theology it is also true that concepts without vision are blind. Systematic theology became blind: above all it lost vision in time – a loss which was to prove particularly disastrous in view of the signs of the time written with large letters on the wall of the era.

Finally, the social dimension was also felt to be an obstacle on the way to a complete scholarly form, although in his early work *Unity in the Church* Johann Adam Möhler insisted that it is not the individual but the community of faith, already invoked in the Letter to the Ephesians, which can be regarded as the complete subject of the knowledge of God.[10] Nevertheless, there was a subjectivistic narrowing down of theological thought. As a result, in the end theological schemes were no longer named after the directions that they took – dialectical, liberal, neo-scholastic, hermeneutic – but rather after their creators: Barth, Bultmann, Guardini, Rahner. They were thus attributed to individual efforts of thought.[11]

The self-correction

As the mention of Möhler shows, however, counter-forces also became active, which worked for a revision of the development that has been described. In fact about the beginning of this century a process began which in the course of a comprehensive self-correction worked to reintroduce the dimensions which had been cast off. This now needs to be sketched in a retrospective direction.

A beginning had to be made with regaining the social sphere, not least because this move was matched by an analogous development in the field of scientific medicine. Whereas the main strand of contemporary theology is still governed by schemes which owe their shape to the unmistakable features of their creators and have their 'seal of approval' in this derivation from an individual way of thinking, in the field of scientific medicine Hans Schaefer, with his concept of a social medicine, worked for the incorporation of social factors into the sphere of medical research and action. In the field of theology it was the political theory developed by Jürgen Moltmann and Johann Baptist Metz which, developing from Latin American liberation theology, started above all with the incorporation of the community into the concept of the subject of faith and thus worked for a 'deprivatization' of theological thought which had been long overdue.[12]

First we have to note a delay in the regaining of the aesthetic dimension, in so far as Odo Marquard countered the thesis of the rebirth of images with the thesis of the anaesthetizing of the present-day world. That makes it all the more important here to recall Martin Deulinger, who was overshadowed by lasting tragedy in his life. He was the first to refer to the value of artistic testimonies of faith in the face of a theology which had become increasingly abstract (Müller-Schwefe).[13] Hans Urs von Balthasar followed in his footsteps with a multi-volume theological aesthetics under the title *The Glory of God*, though in contrast to Deutinger's more comprehensive approach his perspective was restricted to literature.[14] In the meantime there have been clear signs that the distinctive value of the artist's testimony to faith, of which the early church must still have been clearly aware, must be recovered and grounded in the knowledge that the great artists had their own intuitive and invasive grasp of the religious mystery. Consequently their work has its own power of expression, which needs to be noted by theology and preaching. The thesis of anaesthetization could not have been more firmly falsified.

By comparison, the function of a therapeutic theology focussed on regaining the power of healing must first of all be defined in negative terms. It cannot in any way be concerned to win back the territory ceded to scientific medicine and to put itself on the side of the spiritual healers and those who pray for health. That is expressed by a statement which oscillates between regret, wonder and irony: 'The miracles of Jesus have fallen into the hands of the doctors.' Admiring regret and regretful admiration are mixed in this statement, because with the great diastasis, theology has lost one of the prerogatives that Jesus achieved with his life. That on the basis of such spectacular achievements as transplants one can speak of 'miracles' is bound up not least with the thesis developed by Sigmund Freud in his essay on 'Civilization and its Discontents', that modern advanced technology has moved from the side of human beings concerned to ease their existences to that of the dreamers. It has concentrated on the realization of what humankind has dreamed of for millennia: the 'heavenly fire' tamed in nuclear reactors; the journey to the stars achieved in the landings on the moon; and the 'cold heart' (to use Hauff's phrase) which has been realized in transplantation technique. In all these cases utopias have been achieved which resemble the utopia of the kingdom of God anticipated in the miracles of Jesus.[15]

By contrast, the ironic undertone of the statement refers to the effects of the diastasis which are fatal for both sides. These lead to a 'cramping': a cramping of theology so that it becomes objectifying thinking, which can be explained by the effect of Aristotelianism. This turns the mysteries into objects of faith, described in too propositional a way. But that also applies to medicine, which in a quite comparable way must degrade the patient to the 'case' in order to apply its instruments of diagnosis and therapy successfully. In this fashion the doctor who investigates and treats the patient assumes the position of the 'wounded' physician who according to Paracelsus has to empathize with the patient and so share in his suffering in order to be able to heal him. In Jesus description of himself as a 'physician' this is matched by the objection to himself which he makes in the controversy with the visitors to the synagogue in Nazareth, in the call 'Physician, heal yourself' (Luke 4.23).[16]

Anyone who probes the depth of this wounding sees the doctor in a complicated confrontation with death, as in the Grimms' fairy tale *Death the Reaper*. Because of the doctor's successes, Death seems to be engaged in a rearguard action, but at a given time he takes his revenge. This is an exact description of the present conflict. Certainly scientific medicine has not only succeeded in shifting the statistical point of death into the eighth decade, but, even more amazingly, has almost completely put an end to all acute illnesses, including those as devastating as leprosy, cholera and tuberculosis. However, the death which was banished from the world of life has entered it again by the back door, first of all in the form of an illness for which there was not even a name, so that even now it has to be spoken of with the artificial term AIDS. Even more serious is the fact that to the degree that the acute illnesses have been removed, the number of chronically sick who cannot be helped by scientific means has grown to a disturbing degree. By the estimation of the present-day society, focussed on achievement, consumption and enjoyment, the chronically ill are the living dead, since they do not count either as achievers or consumers, and moreover have been made incapable of enjoyment by their illness. Even worse, they themselves regard themselves as dead. For they have lost any feeling of being useful or indispensable for others, or even significant. Being left in the growing solitude of their illness destroys the rest of their feeling of self-worth, so that they seem to themselves to be superfluous, if not a burden on others – people who would be better no longer being there.

The therapy

It is here that the positive contribution of a therapeutic theology can be made: offering meaning in the wilderness of supposed meaninglessness. A work of art can also clarify this task – as the Michelangelo fresco can clarify the idea of God the Creator. In this case the picture is that of the crucifixion on the Isenheim altar. For the gesture of John the Baptist in the scarlet garment of his martyrdom, pointing to the crucified Jesus, conveys a message which can hardly be made in a more striking way. Its simplest rendering is 'Suffering makes sense'. If the loss of the senses ultimately derives from the threat of death, as is shown by consideration of the distress of the chronically sick, the question posed is that of the relationship of Christianity and its theological interpretation to death. Here the answer is that Christianity is the only religion which has dealt with death in its message of the resurrection. But in that case it is clear that the principle of this conquest of death must show itself where the meaningfulness of suffering appears in the direction in which the finger in the Isenheim altarpiece is pointing: to the cross. Just as the threat of death reaches out into the wilderness of meaninglessness, so the embodiment of the fullness of meaning shines out in the death of Jesus on the cross – a death which is accepted in the supreme sense of the word: the love of God which overcomes death.

Over this there are two veils. The first is in the form of the view which can be traced back to the New Testament writings, but not to the relevant statements of Jesus, that Jesus had to die as an expiatory sacrifice for the sins of the world. For the plausibility of this theory of satisfaction, which seems to remove all questions, is overshadowed by the fact that it presupposes a view of God which had clearly been superseded by Jesus. In the central achievement of his life, which shows him to have been the greatest revolutionary in the history of religion, though at the same time the most gentle of all revolutionaries, he had completely blotted out the shadow of wrath and penal justice from the image of God in the religious traditions, including that of his own people. He replaced it with the face of the Father whose love is unconditional. Moreover the doctrine of sacrifice and expiation functionalized the death of Jesus and subjected it to a goal, however lofty. But this has brought home in particular to the philosophy of this century, under the impact of the tremendous harvest which death has reaped in this, the bloodiest era of human history so far, that human death must be thought of and treated purely for itself, because in death it becomes definitively clear what the existence of the dying person was about. To put it another way, death is about the meaning of being human.[17]

Now if this veil of the cross of Jesus is taken away, the meaning of his unfailing trust in God, his mission and the surrender of his life for others spontaneously shines out in it, namely love. Therefore, metaphorically speaking, an invisible sun rose in the night of Golgotha: the sun of the love experienced by Jesus, which points back to his God. This answers both the question of human identity and also the meaning of his suffering – and also, indeed in particular, the meaning of chronic suffering.

The second veil lies over the eyes of those who should have perceived this enlightening answer: the eyes of anxious people. For anxiety is an anticipation of death which is felt every day and therefore, like death itself, is a darkness which does not allow any meaning to appear and be recognized.[18] Now since, as Karl Jaspers said decades ago, the fate of present-day men and women is for their way to be darkened by an 'unprecedented anxiety about life', an authority must be sought which can overcome anxiety.[19] Here too in the broad field of therapies none offers itself as directly as Christianity, which proves itself to be the great religion for overcoming anxiety, in the same way as it takes up the battle with death. In the face of the practice of all the Christian confessions for centuries, which despite all their differences agree that the recalcitrant human being must be driven to accept its offer of salvation with the scourge of the anxiety of sin and hell, that too sounds like a fairy tale. But beyond question one of the secret signs of hope in the present is the fact that – as in the execution machine in Kafka's parable 'In the Penal Colony' – this mechanism has collapsed, so that religious education can no longer be practised by promoting anxiety. It seems that inexorably the centre of Christianity given with what Jesus achieved in his life is establishing itself against all disturbances, even against the effect of an anxiety which shuts off the heavenly light.

Now if the two veils are removed, the only thing that appears from the cross is that for which Jesus lived with the surrender of his whole heart and spirit: unconditional love. And then indeed in the night of Golgotha the sun of the divine love which shines through everything arises. It tells the lonely that they are accepted and have a home; the doubting that they are recognized and understood; the seeking that they have arrived; the anxious that they are safe. And because meaning arises where people are claimed and used, for the chronically ill that means that they are not suffering in vain, because suffering has a meaning. As the great thinker of early Christianity hidden under the name of Dionysius the Areopagite says, God is recognized more through suffering than through research: *non discens, sed patiens divina*.[20]

The practice

When we think of the resistance which Jesus came up against in proclaiming his message of love, which not only (according to John 6.66) led the masses to fall away but ultimately even led to his death, the question of concrete mediation becomes unavoidable. Like other tasks of this magnitude, it can be achieved only by way of co-operation, i.e. in an active community of therapeutic theology and what Bock has called medical 'salutogenesis'. Here theology, recalling the request of the centurion concerned for the life of his servant, 'only speak a word and my servant will be healed' (Matt. 8.8), must reflect primarily on the effective power of the word and the qualities of language, which go far beyond present-day linguistics. For as the result of the narrowing of linguistic to a linguistic analysis which concentrates on originating and transferring information, which does not fully understand its object even by incorporating performative speech-acts (thus Austin),[21] sight is lost of the fact that words can hurt and insult, but can also raise up and comfort. An applied 'theotherapy' must concentrate on this.[22]

Here it is a matter of using convincing language which seeks to make the patients aware of their inner blockages; participative language which seeks to break the spell of their loneliness; uplifting language which seeks to consolidate their feeling of worth which has been attacked; and especially comforting promises, though these of course become effective only on the basis of real empathy and participation.

Here medical support is frequently needed, since the chronically sick are often in such a deep depression that even good talk cannot of itself help them. However, scientific medicine has a number of means – drugs, physiotherapy, psychology and group dynamics – which can be used successfully to break through the barriers of depression. Though the word has to be regarded as a natural medium, in addition the use of other media like pictures and music needs to be considered – here especially we remember David's harp-playing (I Sam. 16.23), which was for therapeutic ends.[23] Over and above the success in healing, however, the decisive question is whether by this means it is possible to rouse in sick persons hope in their healing. For it is not so much the means used as the energies released by faith which bring about relief or even healing. But the decisive shift comes when the sick people are helped to accept their fate and thus themselves. Therefore the programme of therapeutic theology can be summed up in the sentence:

Suffering has meaning!

Translated by John Bowden

Notes

1. For the whole question see my *Theologie als Therapie. Zur Wiedergesinnung einer verlorenen Dimension*, Heidelberg 1985.

2. F. Hahn, *Christologische Hoheitstitel. Ihre Geschichte im frühen Christentum*, Göttingen 1966, 347ff.; C. Schneider, *Geistesgeschichte des antiken Christentums* I, Munich 1954, 724.

3. See J. Gnilka, *Jesus von Nazareth, Botschaft und Geschichte*, Freiburg 1990, 181f., 270f.

4. Ibid., 118–39.

5. See I. Maisch, *Die Heilung des Gelähmten. Eine exegetisch-traditionsgeschichtliche Untersuchung zu Mk 2, 1–12*, Stuttgart 1971.

6. See R. Heinzmann, *Thomas von Aquin*, Heidelberg and Graz 1960, 325–35.

7. I. Kant, *Der Streit der Fakultäten*, Hamburg 1959, 21.

8. K. Löwith, *Vorträge und Aufsätze. Zur Kritik der christlichen Überlieferung*, Stuttgart 1966, 54–96.

9. Cf. C. Tresmontant, *Biblisches Denken und Hellenische Überlieferung*, Düsseldorf 1956, 76f.

10. J. A. Möhler, *Die Einheit in der Kirche*, Tübingen 1843, 100.

11. See J. B. Bauer (ed.), *Entwürfe der Theologie*, Graz 1985.

12. See C. Bussmann, *Befreiung durch Jesus? Die Christologie der Lateinamerikanischen Befreiungstheologie*, Munich 1980, 27.

13. F. Wiedmann, 'Martin Deulinger (1815–1864)', in *Katholische Theologen Deutschlands im 19. Jahrhundert*, II, Munich 1975, 265–92.

14. V. Spangenberg, *Herrlichkeit des Neuen Bundes. Zur Bestimmung des biblischen Begriffs der 'Herrlichkeit' bei Hans Urs von Balthasar*, Tübingen 1993, 4–23.

15. S. Freud, 'Civilization and its Discontents', in *Civilization, Society and Religion*, The Penguin Freud Library 12, Harmondsworth 1991.

16. See U. Busse, *Das Nazareth-Manifest Jesu. Eine Einführung in das Lukanische Jesusbild nach Lk 4, 16–30*, Stuttgart 1977, 38ff.

17. See 'Bindet ihn los! Vom Sinn des Todes Jesu', in my *Glaubensbewährung*, Augsburg 1995, 9–28.

18. See 'Der tägliche Tod: Die Angst', in my *Der Mensch – das uneingelöste Versprechen. Entwurf einer Modellanthropologie*, Düsseldorf 1995, 122–36.

19. K. Jaspers, *Die geistige Situation der Zeit* (1931), Berlin 1971, 55.

20. Ps.-Dionysius the Areopagite, *On the Divine Names*, ch. 2.

21. J. L. Austin, *How to Do Things With Words*, Oxford 1962; see L. Bejerkolm and G. Hornig, *Wort und Handlung. Untersuchungen zur analytischen Religionsphilosophie*, Gütersloh 1966; also my *Menschsein und Sprache*, Salzburg 1989, 67–83.

22. *Theologie als Therapie* (n. 1), 158–63.

23. There are more details in my outline of a media therapy in *Politische Studien* 42, 1991, 61–73.

The Anointing of the Sick: The Oscillation of the Church between Physical and Spiritial Healing

Gisbert Greshake

As far back as we can trace the history of the 'fifth sacrament', it oscillates between the two poles of 'anointing the sick' (with the goal of physical healing or at least the improvement of health) and 'extreme unction' (with the goal of a spiritual healing, namely the forgiveness of sins and preparation for the encounter with God in death). Here both poles have referred and still refer to the basic biblical text, James 5.13ff., but with different interpretations.

The first pole: anointing the sick

The first pole takes up the healing activity of Jesus and his disciples (cf. Mark 6.13) and in this light understands the anointing with oil and prayer in the name of Jesus in James 5 as an effective sign of the healing power of God through the Kyrios. Accordingly at least since the third century the liturgical tradition is attested of the consecration of oil by the bishop.[1] The prayers used here express the fact that through consecration the oil receives the power to bring strengthening and health. The oil consecrated in this way was itself regarded as the 'bearer' of grace, i.e. as a sacramental sign (in the broad sense) which can then be applied not only by those who hold church office but by any giver (it was even possible to anoint oneself). The occasion and object of such an anointing could in principle be 'anything': a headache, a dog-bite, even the slightest sense of being unwell, but of course also more important illnesses. Alongside an anointing proper, people also used the same anointed oil when washing and drinking. In the new significance of being a bearer of

Christ's blessing, the function of oil in antiquity (it was a panacea and food, a giver of light and an apotropaic sign) was preserved. Thus the consecrated oil was also used for exorcistic practices, to some degree as an alternative to pagan magic. It was to provide healing, help and protection against every conceivable damage to the good life. Thus basically oil had a great similarity to what we today understand and use as holy water.[2]

The second pole: 'extreme unction'

The second pole similarly refers to James 5 and does so with greater weight, since the earliest commentary on this passage[3] understands being ill as being a sinner and the presbyteral action as the forgiveness of sins. Accordingly, in the churches of the East the canonical reconciliation of penitents was often associated with a rite of anointing. The understanding of the anointing of the sick (Greek *euchelaion*, literally anointing prayer) in the Eastern churches is stamped with this. To the present day anointing is on the one hand a cure in cases of illness and on the other the completion of penance, not only for the sick but also for those who are physically healthy.[4] Since from the fourth/fifth century onwards canonical repentance was usually postponed to the hour of death because then reconciliation was given without the extremely severe penances, penitential anointing predominantly had its place *in extremis*.

This practice may well have influenced the West also: here from around the time of the Carolingians we observe that anointing is increasingly dominated by the notion of penitence and preparation for death. Moreover because of the exorbitant material contributions required in some places for the gift, which was now reserved for persons holding office in the church to administer, and because of the serious consequences if one were to recover (those whose senses had been 'consecrated' by the anointing had henceforth to shun many earthly pleasures), anointing was put off until the last moment. So more and more it was practised only on the fatally ill and the dying. When a specific theology of the sacraments (in the sense of the 'seven sacraments') was worked out in the eleventh/twelfth centuries, there was no problem in including such an anointing; indeed this even gave it a special dignity. In the words of Thomas Aquinas: 'This sacrament is the last and as it were all-embracing sacrament of the whole spiritual way of salvation, through which the human being is prepared to participate in the divine glory. Hence it is also called Extreme Unction' (*ScG* IV, 73). 'It blots out the remnants of sin and prepares people for the final glory' (*STh* III 65, 1c).

Thus the two poles of this sacrament which present themselves almost as alternatives are called anointing of the sick *or* Extreme Unction, physical healing *or* spiritual salvation. Are these arguments or criteria for one or the other alternative?

Wrong ways in scholasticism?

A favourite argument for depicting 'Extreme Unction' as outdated and inadequate is that the mediaeval understanding that the sacrament brings about *spiritual* healing and *spiritual* salvation is simply a consequence both of actual (perverted) practice at the time and of a defective historical knowledge about the original therapeutic anointing of the sick.[5] But this argument passes over reality: the scholastic understanding is more the result of 1. a deeper view of sacramentality and 2. the inner 'theological logic' of a 'sacramental world' marked by the seven sacraments.

1. The scholastics arrived at a deeper understanding of what a sacrament (now deliberately opposed to a sacramental) is: it is of the nature of the seven sacraments that in word and sign God's *unconditional* promise is given to be present and effective in a particular human situation with his grace. W. Simonis rightly observes: 'Of course a healing of sickness can also be termed grace; however, it is not *this* grace that is the "content" of the anointing of the sick, but the . . . strictly supernatural grace of "eternal life" with God . . . Were earthly healing the significance of this sacrament, then it would not be a "visible sign of *invisible grace*" but a visible sign of a reality which again became *visible*.'[6] Furthermore it would not be an *unconditional* promise, since in most cases, or at least in very many cases, the anointing of the sick would be an ineffective sign, as very often healing or improvement did not take place.

2. For scholastic theology the seven sacraments are not just 'some' holy and hallowing signs but promises of salvation with which the decisive points where individual and social human life crystallize are very closely connected.[7] Such a crystallization point is also, and indeed specially, the situation of the human being 'in the face of death', in which a sacrament is the preparation for receiving the divine glory. One could almost say that were there not such a sacrament, a decisive human situation would remain sacramentally 'unoccupied'.[8] But the question arises: with this scholastic understanding is not the previous exegetical and liturgical tradition – as E. Lengeling observes – 'to an amazing degree ignored or even violated in favour of a speculative delight in systems'?[9] By no means.

First, the scholastics were completely orientated on a therapeutic anointing practised in early times. Thus e.g. Petrus Cantor writes in a discussion of Mark 6.13: 'About which anointing does the Lord speak here? Extreme Unction? . . . No, the Lord speaks of anointings which were performed with chrism or another holy oil and with which the sick were healed . . . But because of misuse the habit of anointing the sick for the purpose of healing (*ungendi infirmos causa salutis consequende*) soon became lost.'[10] Moreover, for the scholastics such anointings did not have the character of a sacrament, but of a sacramental.

Thus, as W. Simonis observes in a vivid but probably not inaccurate way, in the scholastic theology of the sacraments there took place

> nothing less than a rejection of the idea that the anointing of the sick served for the restoration of *earthly* health. To call *this* notion the more holistic understanding, encompassing this world and the world to come . . . may well be simply a gross misunderstanding. It was not an expression of a holistic understanding but a piece of quackery from late antiquity. Rather, a holistic understanding first appears where the phenomenon of an earthly having-to-die is taken seriously in the whole of its radical nature, and precisely this phenomenon of nothingness, final threat and the fragility of body and soul 'in this world' is *nevertheless* believed in as a sign of the completion of the whole person 'in the world to come'.[11]

But neither in the view of the time nor from a present-day perspective did the scholastic interpretation set itself speculatively above exegesis. Let us take James 5, the basic text. First of all, here we have a patient who is confined to bed, and is therefore *seriously* ill, so that he has to have the presbyters called; they come so that he may receive 'salvation' (*sozein*) through their action. What is important is the interpretation of this concept[12] is that the Letter of James has a markedly eschatological tenor and that the fourfold use of the term *sozein* probably fits in best here; in other words this is salvation in the final, eschatological sense. The promise of the 'raising up' (*egeirein*) of the sick person probably also corresponds to this. Even if we note the broad biblical significance of *egeirein*, we must not overlook the fact that for Christians there is also an echo of the resurrection. So Grillmeier rightly asked: 'Did not the recipients or readers of the Letter of James first read this [new, peculiarly Christian tenor] out of it?'[13]

The exegete Gerhard Lohfink has shown from quite a different direction, namely the original significance of baptism, how the traditional conception 'fits' with exegesis: baptism 'cannot be understood at all without its basic eschatological structure. It is given with a view to the imminent end.'[14] Now *de facto* this significance retreated in the reshaping of primitive Christian eschatology. However – Lohfink observes – 'in the course of time a large part of the basic eschatological orientation of baptism seems to have gone over to the sacrament of the anointing of the sick . . . The seriously sick person was anointed and sealed for the end.' So Lohfink asks: 'If there is horror today at the development of the anointing of the sick into a "sacrament for the dying" and it is seen as a serious error, with the result that the connections between the anointing of the sick and the sacrament of the dying are again deliberately being relaxed or even broken, where within the economy of all the sacraments is the place at which the sealing for the end is really expressed?'[15] Such reflections fit very precisely with the state of the problem in scholastic theology, for which the *anthropological* 'location' of the 'fifth sacrament' is the 'view of the end'. As for the *christological* context of this sacrament, the scholastic solution similarly corresponds to the New Testament basis. In the words of Simonis, the death of Christ on the cross is

> the primal sacramental model of Christian dying; and the sacrament of the anointing of the sick brings out that the illness and dying of Christians is also discipleship of Christ, and that to this degree it supplements what is still lacking in the whole of the body of Christ (see Col. 1.24) . . . [On this line] the anointing of the sick is the confession of the believing church that the same Spirit which raised Christ also makes Christians' illness and dying, i.e. their earthly end, a sign of consummation.[16]

What becomes of the perspective of physical healing?

The scholastic theology of the sacraments – at any rate the theology of the so-called seven sacraments which is historically first and fundamental – firmly put the fifth sacrament in the sphere of spiritual healing and spiritual salvation. But its medical and therapeutic function was by no means overlooked. On the contrary. Thomas Aquinas gives a fundamentally positive answer to the question whether physical healing is part of the effect of this sacrament; however, he locates this answer in the *primarily* spiritual sense of the sacrament: God 'never produces the secondary effect [bodily healing] unless it furthers the primary effect [spiritual salvation]. Therefore bodily healing does not always result from the sacrament, but only when it furthers spiritual healing. Then, however, the sacrament always produces that, supposing that the recipient does not pose any obstacle' (*STh suppl.* 30, 2c). Moreover this integrative view also finds its way into the texts of the Council of Trent: the sacrament of the sick raises up the sick person 'so that he bears the burdens . . . of the illness more easily and sometimes achieves bodily healing if that is useful for the salvation of the soul' (*DS* 1694ff.).

Thus the medical-therapeutic aspect is integrated into the sacrament at a secondary stage. However, it does not follow from this that the church has pushed Jesus' commandment to heal the sick into second place. To exaggerate, one could even say that to the degree that the fifth sacrament was understood as being primarily orientated on spiritual healing and spiritual salvation, an increasing network of therapeutic action by the church was developed in hospitals, homes for the handicapped and nursing institutions, in which not only the routine of the day and the way in which the sick were cared for but also the action of physical healing, even to the area of internal arrangements (cf. e.g. the Hôtel de Dieu in Beaune), stood in the sphere of faith.

The further development and its problems

Whereas the statements of traditional theology and the directives of the magisterium attempted to integrate bodily and spiritual healing, individual theologians in the nineteenth century went a step further by understanding the fifth sacrament in terms of only one of its poles, as a 'sacrament of dedication to death'.[17] This had the practical consequence that at least since then it was understood and practised *only* as a sacrament of the dying. Occasionally the canon lawyers said that the criterion of the danger of death governed not only whether the sacrament was permissible, but even whether it was valid. Vatican II (not without objections from a few [especially Germany] bishops) introduced a clear emphasis which countered this: ' "Extreme Unction", which may also and more fittingly be called "Anointing of the Sick", is not a sacrament for those only who are at the point of death. Hence, as soon as anyone of the faithful begins to be in danger of death from sickness or old age, the fitting time for him to receive this sacrament has certainly already arrived' (SC 73). This tendency is further reinforced in Paul VI's post-conciliar Apostolic Constitution of 1972: the designation Extreme Unction and the reference to the life-threatening nature of the illness are avoided, though at the same time – in an ambiguous way – the corresponding statements of the Council of Trent are repeated. All in all, in fact 'the reorientation of the sacrament of Extreme Unction so that it becomes the sacrament of the anointing of the sick was at first only cautiously given official legitimation at the Second Vatican Council; it was completed all the more consistently in the post-conciliar documents'.[18] Furthermore the new Ritual emphasized the solemn character of the anointing of the sick and therefore also provided for communal celebrations for all people who were merely 'in some way' older. A series of national Rituals go one step further in their practical instructions; influenced by some historians of liturgy with their extremely one-sided view of the practice of anointing in the early church, which has often not been reflected on hermeneutically, they emphasize the 'medicinal' character of the sacrament, relate it to any form of illness,[19] and thus seek to detach it completely from the dimensions 'in the face of death' (or even 'in the face of the boundaries of life in death').[20] Here the pendulum has swung completely away from the understanding of the fifth sacrament as a 'sacrament of dedication to death' to the healing hoped for from the sacrament with emphasis on physical healing or at least improvement (though of course without excluding spiritual salvation).[21] What is to be said about the present trend?

First of all the history of all the sacraments shows that the church has the competence within a certain framework to mark out more precisely the 'scope' of a sacrament. This can be seen particularly clearly in the case of this sacrament 'between' anointing of the sick and Extreme Unction. Nevertheless, it seems to me that questions need to be asked about the present swing of the pendulum:

1. Can one elevate one period of church history, the early period, with its therapeutic practice, so exclusively to become the norm for this sacrament, as a series of liturgical scholars do, at the same time filtering out elements which do not fit, like the fact of a 'penitential unction at the end' or a failure to observe the very unspecific use of consecrated oil?

2. What is the hermeneutical significance of the fact that in the rise of a specific theology of the sacraments, the fifth sacrament was counted among the seven sacraments not as the anointing of the sick but as Extreme Unction, and as such constituted the sacramental 'cosmos' (i.e. the ordering between the sacraments and their relationship to human life)?

3. Is there not a danger of succumbing to dangerous fashions in both failing to note the penitential character (which after all is a theme in James 5 [the forgiveness of sins] and has a long tradition) and above all in cutting out the situation of death? Thus sociologists are already asking whether in a society which represses death the new emphasis has not brought relief from 'an unpopular task, namely being a messenger of death'.[22] Indeed, is not perhaps this circumstance even the 'vehicle' – usually unconscious – for the present swing of the pendulum?

4. Furthermore, is the alternative 'physical or spiritual healing' (which was given to me in the formulation of the subject for this article) appropriate?

Attempt at a synthesis

In Holy Scripture, sickness, sin and death form a single syndrome: in severe illness or advanced old age death casts its shadow forward, and in both, the disintegration of creation ultimately caused by sin is experienced in a concrete and deeply inward sense. The result is that the whole of the person is shaken. Men and women react with anxiety, hopelessness and despair or with impatience and rebellion. In this situation the reception of the fifth sacrament (like any other sacrament) represents an embodiment of the saving promise and saving presence of Christ. Here the *specific* element of this sacrament is encounter with the 'healing' but also the 'suffering and glorified Lord' to whom 'the whole church commends those who are ill, that he may raise them up and save them', together with the invitation and possibility to 'unite themselves freely to the passion and death of Christ . . . and so contribute to the good of the People of God' (*Lumen Gentium* 11). Thus this sacrament is in a sense the 'renewal of baptism' in a situation which confronts people with frontiers of their life with which they themselves cannot cope. Such a view in principle goes beyond the alternative of 'anointing the sick or Extreme Unction', 'physical or spiritual salvation or healing'. For in the encounter with Christ actualized in the reality of baptism, a renewal of faith, hope and love takes place. Now it is the *hope* in faith and love which relates not only to the 'last and final', but also to the 'penultimate and provisional'. Karl Barth puts it very well: 'The promised future is not only that of the day of the Lord at the end of all days, but because it is the end and goal of all days, it is also today and tomorrow.'[23] God's promised salvation does not just reach people at the end, but is now already effective in small fragments. Now already God's last future is outlined in signs. Therefore the content of the Christian hope is not just the 'great hope' but also the many 'small hopes', signs in which the ultimate shows itself in advance and is a motivation towards the great hope.[24] This in particular was also the significance of the symbolic actions of Jesus, especially his healings of the sick: he did not make the world a paradise already, but did signs of hope so that the great hope of the kingdom could come into being. So if the fifth sacrament communicates hope in faith and love in the face of death, it also includes signs of hope which can be experienced.

That does not just mean that in the sacrament the church asks for the healing of the seriously ill or for an overcoming of the crisis of ageing for the very old – at least for a few years.[25] It means far more: that Christian hope will grasp the sick and the old in their unity of body and soul and provide tangible help, so that with strength, patience and trust they may withstand the crisis of their illness, the decay of life and the threat of death. The 'last' hope (for spiritual salvation) and hopes for help in serious illness (physical salvation) are therefore not unrelated, but are strictly related: in the sign of hope 'in the face of death' people can experience that they are called to the 'last' hope and enabled to have such a hope. A new integration of the physical and the spiritual aspects can be found along this line, not very removed from the high-scholastic solution which emphasizes the priority of spiritual healing and communicates physical healing (which in any case in modern times has 'emancipated' itself as a separate medical sphere) by means of spiritual salvation and spiritual healing.

Translated by John Bowden

Notes

1. Cf. e.g. Hippolytus, *Apostolic Tradition* 5.

2. By contrast, in the early church holy water was used more for lustrative purposes.

3. Origen, *Hom. in Lev.* 2, 4.

4. Cf. E. Mélia, 'Le sacrement des malades. Un témoignage orthodoxe', *Présences* 90, 1965, 133–42; R. Hotz, *Sakramente – im Wechselspiel zwischen Ost und West*, Zurich, etc. 1979, 197, 254f.

5. This is a favourite commonplace remark, which can be found for example in H. Vorgrimler, *Busse und Krankensalbung*, HDG IV, 3, Freiburg im Breisgau 1978, 222. Present-day liturgical scholars in particular cannot talk enough about the 're-functioning', the 'forgetting', the 'narrowing' of the original sacraments of the sick with the aim of therapeutic healing. See e.g. R. Kaczynski, 'Neubesinnung auf ein "Vergessenes" Sakrament', *ThPQ* 121, 1973, 349; A. Knauber, 'Krankensalbung', *Handbuch der Pastoraltheologie* IV, Freiburg im Breisgau 1969, 147, 163; E. J. Lengeling, 'Todesweihe oder Krankensalbung?', *Liturgisches Jahrbuch* 21, 1971, 212f.

6. W. Simonis, *Glaube und Dogma der Kirche: Lobpreis seiner Herrlichkeit*, St Ottilien 1995, 540.

7. Cf. Thomas Aquinas, *STh* III, 65, 1.

8. The viaticum cannot take over this role. Cf. G. Greshake, 'Letzte Ölung – Krankensalbung – Tauferneuerung angesichts des Todes?', in R. Schulte (ed.), *Leiturgia – Koinonia – Diakonia, FS Kardinal Fritz König*, Vienna, Freiburg and Basel 1980, 121–68.

9. Cf. Lengeling, 'Todesweihe' (n. 5), 213.

10. Quoted from H. Weisweiler, 'Das Sakrament der Letzten Ölung in den systematischen Werken der ersten Frühscholastiker', *Scholastik* 7, 1932, 327f. – Petrus's pupil Robert de Courçon also knows different anointings. Similarly Thomas Aquinas knows of anointings with oil for the sick by laity. He comments that their functions were not sacramental (*quod illae functiones non erant sacramentales*, *STh*, Suppl. 31, 1 ad 2.

11. Simonis, *Glaube und Dogma* (n. 6), 541.

12. This is pointed out by A. Grillmeier, 'Das Sakrament der Auferstehung', *GuL* 34, 1961, 329.

13. Ibid., 330. But that would be very much in line with the first theological commentary on James 5 in Origen, according to which eschatological salvation and resurrection are promised in the anointing.

14. G. Lohfink, 'Der Ursprung der christlichen Taufe', *ThQ* 156, 1976, 52.

15. Ibid., 53.

16. Simonis, *Glaube und Dogma* (n. 6), 540.

17. Thus M. J. Scheeben, *Mysterien des Christentums*, ed. V. J. Hofer, Freiburg 1941, 475; H. Schell, *Katholische Dogmatik*, III, 2, Paderborn 1893, 614–40.

18. A. Moos, ' "Krankensalbung" oder "Letzte Ölung"?', in H. Becker, B. Einig and P.-O. Ullrich (eds.), *Im Angesicht des Todes*, II, St Ottilien 1987, 793. However, to think, as Moos does, that here the church has spoken its 'last word' fails to recognize the fundamental historicity of sacramental practice and overlooks the fact that the radical steps towards detaching the fifth sacrament from any relationship with death has not been taken by the church's magisterium but by particular theologians.

19. Cf. e.g. G. Davanzo, 'L'unzione degli infermi', *EphLit* 89, 1975, 333, who proposes as a principle '(The recipient of the anointing is) someone who thinks that he or she is ill'.

20. R. Kaczynski, 'Die Feier der Krankensakramente. Für eine pastorale Praxis entsprechend der liturgischen Ordnung', *Ikaz* 12, 1983, 423–36.

21. This new trend also offers advantages for ecumenical dialogue. See K. Lehmann and W. Pannenberg (eds.), *Confessions of the Reformation Era. Do They Still Divide?*, Philadelphia 1989, 138f.: 'The Protestant churches, too, are firmly convinced that the pastoral promise made with prayer, which can be visibly combined with a sign of blessing, can give the sick person the trustworthy certainty of faith that . . . in Jesus Christ God has given us a physician . . . whose spirit can make us whole in body and soul.'

22. J. Schmied, 'Einstellung zu Tod und Unsterblichkeit', in *Stichwort Tod*, ed. G. Gebhardt, Frankfurt 1979, 46.

23. K. Barth, *Church Dogmatics* IV/1, Edinburgh 1956, 120f.

24. For the terminology 'great hope' – 'small hopes', cf. ibid.

25. However, the hearing of prayer cannot be the real intention of the sacrament. One need only reflect how much being sick or healthy is 'relativized' in a good sense in the tradition of the church. For the *Exercises* of Ignatius of Loyola it is even a criterion for 'indifference': '*Ut non velimus ex parte nostra magis sanitatem quam infirmitatem*' (That for our part we do not want health more than infirmity) (no. 23).

Recent Developments in the Anointing of the Sick

Kristiaan Depoortere

Practical theology, more than other disciplines, writes from a particular context. Where theology touches on the actual texture of faith communities, differences come to light. Therefore this article does not offer any solution for just any context. Scholarship requires that we make clear that we write from a particular situation.

This article is situated in Flanders in Belgium, until 1960 an almost homogeneous Catholic region, but now as strongly secularized as the whole of north-west Europe. But the Catholic institutions and organization remain exceptionally strong – also because of a redefinition of their basic values: youth and adult movements, a Christian insurance company, a trade union, a political party, and so on. This results in paradoxes: in 1995 more than 75% of young people studied at Catholic educational institutions; 41% of general hospitals and 88% of psychiatric hospitals were associated with a Christian parent organization. However, at the same time participation in the weekly eucharist has declined between 1967 and 1995 from 52% to 15.2%; the number of church marriages from 91.8% to 54.4%. In health care in almost every hospital there is a permanent, salaried Catholic pastoral ministry. In Christian hospitals the aim is for a full-time person for every 150 to 200 beds. In practice the pastoral ministry consists of a small team of a priest and laity with theological training. In the parishes very few laity are involved in a professional association. Priests and volunteers care for the sick. Outside a sporadic communal celebration, most parish priests have little experience of the anointing of the sick. Sick people are quickly taken to hospitals. This article draws mainly on pastoral practice in hospitals and not on the parishes. The picture of the patient presented to us here is that of someone who is seriously ill, who stays in a hospital for some time, and is in a position to communicate. The options here are somewhat one-sided.

If there were no limit to the length of articles in this journal, I would like to have focussed on the period between the seventh and the ninth centuries. It would emerge from that how close is the link between the form given to anointing with the 'tear of the olive tree' and the evolution of 'sacramental' reconciliation. In the same connection the priest becomes the exclusive minister in the anointing of the sick and this turns into the anointing of the dying, with very explicit attention to spiritual salvation and the forgiveness of sins. The *poenitentia ad mortem* forces the anointing to become *unctio ad mortem*. Secondly, I would have wanted to indicate in this historical survey how the narrowing of the anointing of the sick to the sacrament of the dying was contested through all the following centuries. Pastors, theologians and council fathers (e.g. Trent) argued for the anointing of the *sick*, with an explicit prayer for integral healing, i.e. healing of the body as well.

However, we must move to the present situation, around thirty years after Vatican II. At that council 'extreme unction' again became the anointing of the sick, not without some compromises. The Council wanted an encouraging sacramental gesture for seriously ill people: that they would be saved (*salvare*) and rise (*allevare*) in the most integral meaning of those words. However, in the past thirty years it has proved that the change of meaning has penetrated only to a minority.[1] Why is that? Over the past decades shifts have taken place in health care at the medical and pastoral levels. Our reflection starts there. Meanwhile theological thought about sacraments has also developed. After we have sketched out that development we shall bring the two series of shifts together and ask what is to be done. Should more attempts be made to bring home to the faithful the option taken by Vatican II, or should another way be adopted because the anointing of the *sick* perhaps overlooks a number of anthropological facts? Here we shall throw up a number of ideas for discussion.

Shifts in health care

As the standard of living rises, people live longer . . . and they are often also sick for longer. Often the lengthening of life is also the lengthening of suffering. Certainly, the analgesic effect of drugs can be separated more and more effectively from their anaesthetic effect, allow people to suffer less and yet remain as conscious and as capable of communication as possible. But that often means that people are confronted more sharply with questions about life and death and with anxiety. Therefore an ongoing revision of the relationship between the curing and the caring dimensions of health care are needed. The caring (total care of the patient) must keep pace with the rapid progress in curing, directed towards the restoration of (bodily) health.

In this context, Dr Cicely Saunders, on the basis of an expressly Christian inspiration, took the initiative in palliative care. Starting from the reality of total pain, palliative care tries to offer an integrating answer at the medical, psychological, social and religious levels. Thus palliative care as a mentality is the support and complement to curing. In the terminal phase, when the curing ceases, total care takes over. It is not surprising that in a palliative context new symbols and rituals are discovered in the process of acceptance and in working through mourning, like carefully closing the eyes of a dead person, or handing over the wedding ring to the surviving partner. Because symbols and rituals bring together different levels of being, they are particularly suited to signify total pain. Art therapists who help to give expression to what cannot be said are attached to some palliative centres.[2]

In the spread of the palliative concept of care, the original, explicitly Christian, inspiration of Dame Cicely Saunders has developed into a broad attention to 'spirituality', a kind of greatest common denominator of all religions. Of course that is also very important, but it is very much open to question how most people are served by this. Do the patients still get support for their specific religious need? Doesn't the word 'spirituality' rather reflect the *à la carte* belief of those who look after them?[3]

Pastoral support in health care has also changed deeply. The decline in the number of priests has played a role here. The reintroduction of the permanent diaconate has not helped much. In the first place the development of the diaconate is liturgical. If mission in the charitable sector had been emphasized more strongly, perhaps more deacons would have begun to work in health care. Then the question of the minister in the anointing of the sick would have been unavoidable. Now usually laity work together with priests in the pastoral ministries. For them, too, after the Vatican Instruction on the Collaboration of Non-Ordained Faithful in the Priestly Ministry (15 August 1997), the official leeway is very restricted. Lay people bear different names, like 'pastoral workers', 'pastoral helpers'. They receive very different mandates from the bishop, not necessarily with a liturgical appointment, in more or less agreement between the directors of hospitals and the episcopal vicar in charge of charitable work. The collaboration between a man (usually older and ordained) and a woman (younger and lay) sometimes unexpectedly opens up complementary perspectives. But here too there are problems because the division of responsibility is unclear and views of the church, sacraments and the pastorate contrast greatly.

Often the pastoral workers have meanwhile made the obstacle a springboard and opened up new spheres of work in supporting the sick in faith. To put it in the form of an antithesis: 'In the case of priests (with a classical theological training) a sacrament sometimes offers the occasion for a conversation; in pastoral workers (whose training is more relational) a conversation sometimes comes to be concentrated in a sacrament.' However, this succinct wording reveals a basic difference in approach. We shall return to that in our excursus on sacramental theology.

It is obvious that the question of the minister in the anointing of the sick explicitly emerges here. Some (conferences of) bishops introduce creative tensions in order to do justice to both the standpoint of church law and the concrete work situation. In 1993, with episcopal approval, the Dutch National Council for Liturgy published an official order: *Praying with the Dying*. It is a service book for blessing the dying, though not with the viaticum, which both priests and pastoral workers can use.[4]

It is becoming increasingly difficult to explain why pastoral workers may provide complete support and counsel in faith but not its consummation in the sacrament. The question is acute for priests. Many worry about the validity of the sacrament if their non-ordained colleagues perform a kind of anointing: 'With an invalid sacrament you are deceiving the sick . . .' However, some priests feel that their own identity is also questioned if their non-ordained colleagues do not anoint. It is theologically clear, but existentially they feel that they are 'reduced to ministers of the sacrament', since pastoral workers are doing the most 'attractive' work, namely giving support in the faith. However, more recently, direct questions are also being asked by the health authorities. Some think that the requests of patients – even requests for the anointing of the sick – must be met, even if the diocese can no longer provide a hospital chaplain; even if no priest can be called from a neighbouring parish.

But what does the believing patient require? As I have already remarked, for the majority of the sick, the anointing of the sick has remained 'extreme unction'. The declining church membership and a school catechesis which did not pay very much attention to sacraments and liturgy are important factors here. Or is there more? Has the Vatican II view of the anointing of the sick taken sufficient account of all kinds of anthropological demands? Doesn't the stubborn association of anointing and dying mean that the sick want to reserve that gesture for the last moment? Both the question of the minister in the anointing of the sick and the question whether Vatican II adopted the right option with the anointing of the sick call for an injection of theology.

Towards a development of sacramentality?

Nowadays more attention needs to be paid to the spread of sacramentality, but the term is used in very different senses.[5] This is not the place to go more deeply into the debate. So I shall simply refer briefly to three authors who help our reflections.

On symbols and sacraments, Leonardo Boff writes: 'The world is not divided into immanence and transcendence. There is an intermediate form, the transparency which takes both the immanence and the transcendence into itself . . . Transparency means that the transcendent makes itself present in the immanent and that the latter becomes transparent to the reality of the former. The transcendence that breaks open within the immanent transforms the immanent and makes it transparent.'[6] If we juggle with this meaning, it becomes: 'All of this earthly reality, and certainly all that is love, however human, can become transparent, an icon of the divine.' François-Xavier Durrwell clarifies the question how this process of becoming transparent develops. In his book about the eucharistic presence he says that the decisive factor is the epiclesis.[7] It is by the invocation of the Spirit that the immanent becomes transparent. Here the human does not lose anything of its riches. On the contrary, the world attains its highest power of expression by the indwelling of the Spirit. In connection with the eucharist, the Spirit releases all the potentialities of bread. This bread does not just satisfy physical hunger, but also the deepest hunger for meaning and life. Bread becomes 'breader' and 'breadest', bread in the superlative, so totally transparent that it becomes real presence. Those who feed on this 'breadest' become more and more human, more and more transparent, on the way to the consummation of their humanness. The third author, Louis-Marie Chauvet, says the same thing in three short sentences: 'The "place" of the theological is the anthropologal. The most spiritual is given in the most physical. Isn't that what sacraments confirm?'[8]

These three authors introduce valuable elements for a renewed theology of the sacraments. By that in the first place I mean a theology of the sacraments which is rooted in life and starts from the valuable things that take place there. For a believer, God – since in Christ and in the Spirit God breaks through all the particularistic bounds of people, race and view of life – is at work incognito in the small, daily story of human beings with one another and in the great history of humankind. God struggles with them against meaninglessness and disaster. For health care this means a revaluation of all that is done in love for a sick person, no matter by whom and on what inspiration. God gives signs of life through people, unseen, unrealized, in operations, in combatting pain, during therapy, in examining the conditions for repayment by the insurance company, in looking after the family, in listening to questions about meaning.

In the context of belief this discrete divine presence is sometimes brought to light in passing: the whispering of God's name, a crucifix, a visit to the sick person in the name of the parish, a word of farewell: 'I shall be thinking of you again this evening', the laying on of hands and a blessing. These little rituals used to be called sacramentals. We can use the word again, provided that it does not have the meaning of 'extra' or 'what doesn't quite reach the level of a sacrament'. It is precisely the other way round. Sacramentals are the soil, the breeding ground from which sacraments grow. They are also more than preparations for the sacraments. In a sense they are the ministry of the word which goes with them. They also prevent sacramental gestures from deteriorating into magical signs, if they lose a link with ordinary life and with concrete human contributions.

Sacraments in the strict sense – in a certain sense a third level – are no longer 'passing' ritualizations. In sacraments people stand still. They simply want to bear witness to one another of their love, give eucharist, celebrate reconciliation. Sacraments are an official seal on a process which goes on for a long time, first incognito, then symbolized in passing and now explicitly confirmed. In such a sealing an authorized representative of God and the believing community functions. Such a representative has direct roots in the New Testament.

The sacramental sealing – like a seal on a charter – has three dimensions. First it is authentication: all the previous care of the sick was authentic work. There God gave a sign of life incognito.

This authentication takes place by explicit naming. That is the second significance of healing. The incognito God *speaks*. He speaks in the word of scripture at the anointing of the sick and in the gesture of anointing. Naming his name 'does' something. It completes it and brings it to fullness. Naming his name socalizes: God's name can be heard by all the carers present. Calling on God also personalizes, for he is spoken of over this particular sick person: 'You too, you above all now, are bound up with God in your situation of suffering.'

Finally, the sacramental sealing is a sending. That is the third significance of the seal on a charter. This sending is ethical, even now: 'Be a sign of hope.' There are sick people who understand the art of encouraging their visitors. So sacraments again end up in sacramentals. But the deeper sending is eschatological. The sacramental anointing sets the two preceding aspects in an 'already and not yet' movement. The care of the sick which is declared authentic is a first step on the way to God who is 'all in all'. The consummation is a consummation in embryo, not as a full-grown reality. Invocation implies vocation; calling on God by name in a sacrament means being called and sent. The sick, too, are sent, and live on the way to consummation, redemption and resurrection, with an open future.

Developing the content of sacramentality in this way – from daily life to explicit rite – also includes a liturgical development of different moments of experience. We shall be returning to that shortly. But it also implies the fluent collaboration of various pastors. It is not concerned with undermining the distinct nature of the ordained and authorized representative. But distinctiveness is something different from cumulation. If a woman, in a long series of conversations with a woman pastoral worker in a psychiatric ward, has haltingly come to talk about her abortion, must one then require this confession to be repeated in detail to a strange priest as a *conditio sine qua non* for sacramental absolution? Here the sacrament as sealing becomes concrete. Sometimes a second confession is therapeutically useful. Sometimes it is nothing but humiliation. Should the pastoral worker and the penitent together make a penitential journey to a neighbouring church, where the priest is waiting and leads her into the church, lays hands on her in (telling) silence, gives forgiveness and offers the eucharist? Doesn't this honour both the 'authority' of the priest as 'sealer' and the talents of the supportive pastoral worker, and above all doesn't it show much understanding of the repentant sinner?

But what can such a development of sacramental reality mean for the anointing of the sick?

Between fact and dream: liturgical support for the sick today

At first sight the liturgical framework relating to the sick according to Vatican II seems rich and coherent: first the sacrament of reconciliation, then the anointing of those who are seriously weak or gravely ill, and finally the viaticum for the dying. The recent 'blessing of a dying person' mentioned above fits perfectly into this framework. Emergencies apart, it really poses no problems of ministry. If one arranges the anointing in a timely way, there is time enough to call a priest.

However, on closer examination, there are problems at every stage of this scheme. The sacrament of reconciliation is undergoing a severe crisis in the West. Even many practising Catholics no longer ever make a personal confession. So it is not obvious that they will resume this when they are seriously ill. As for a request for anointing, the criticism has been heard that this fits perfectly into the framework of the taboo about death. Indeed, just a little ill-will is enough to point out that the word 'death' occurs in the order of service for the anointing of a sick person only with reference to Christ. According to this criticism an anointing when there is no danger to life – which sometimes evolves into a 'celebration of the fourth age' – succeeds in avoiding a personal confrontation with mortality. At the theological level some writers point out that the eschatological dimension of Christian faith does not score highly today. But such an evasion of death in the first person does not really satisfy people. Precisely for that reason the renewal of Vatican II fails in precisely the same way as that of Trent on this point: because anthropological requirements are overlooked. People are asking vitally and viscerally for a rite of transition, certainly for the last passage. Too early an anointing robs them of this. People do not want to be anointed unless they themselves – or their families – really feel that it is now or never.

But according to Vatican II is the viaticum the sacrament of the dying? Theologically that fits: the best is saved for last, namely food for the way to the other side. But in our Christian hospitals many believers communicate twice a week. So at an anthropological level the supreme sacrament does not work as a ritual of transition. Not to mention the many medical and practical problems around communion for the dying.

And what about the blessing of dying people? However well-intentioned and however rich in meaning, as a rite of passage this is too verbal and too bleak: there is no substance. And would this rite have been invented if pastoral workers were allowed to administer the anointing of the sick?

Where do we go from here?

I am not arguing for the reintroduction of extreme unction, but for an anointing of the sick which can function effectively as a transitional rite. I would locate this option within a global pastoral strategy of a developed sacramentality. Here are some ideas – more questions than answers.

1. The continuing (or growing) dissociation between faith and healing is a cause for anxiety. We often talk about the healing power of faith, but the books about it are either anthologies of completely miraculous events or merely a transformation of faith into psychotherapy. What is the healing power of sacramental grace? This is an absorbing and urgent area for further investigation.

2. The actual vacuum in the forgiveness of sins is disturbing. As long as people are healthy they may perhaps succeed in putting questions of guilt on one side. That is no longer possible on a sick bed. Real and delusory questions of guilt come flooding in to sick people, certainly if there is not much time left for 'growing towards forgiveness'. Here too a creative collaboration is needed between the humane sciences and religion, between psychotherapy and support in the faith. It would be good if here the liberating message for the penitent stood in the foreground – in line with the example that I gave earlier – and not primarily legal prescriptions. Precisely in the content of the forgiveness of sins, at the beginning of this article I wanted to focus on the eighth and ninth centuries, when there was also such a ritual vacuum. At that time – and again now – this meant that care of the terminally ill had to pay acute attention to questions of guilt. Was the link between the anointing of the sick and the forgiveness of sins then not so random at the moment when dying in the first person became a possibility?

3. In health care, where sick people all too often are fragmented depending on their symptoms and people are isolated from their milieu, an integrating approach is necessary. Pastoral work brings about associations and draws ever wider spirals. The first is within the hospital, so that pastoral care is closely related to palliative care and integrated nursing. The time when a hospital chaplain simply went the rounds is over. Pastors are members of teams and work together closely with the social and the psychological services; if they are allowed to, they share in the briefings of the divisions, and have a contribution of their own to make about the 'whole' sick person. A second spiral links the sick with their families. Often the pastor can bring about reconciliation here. A third spiral brings the sick in contact with their faith communities or parishes. A fourth link connects the sick with God. In the Jewish–

Christian tradition, pastoral work involves making connections and establishing bonds.

4. Making a link with God begins with sensitive listening – being close and offering support – but it also includes speaking. Not all the 'Why?' questions asked by sick people are just a cry for people to be near. Some sick people ask for an understandable explanation and clarification of their situation. So great attention must be paid to the training of hospital chaplains to put them above the level of professional companions. But their spiritual training is just as important. They must help the sick with prayer and thus put them in contact with the One who remains, even if they go away. A broad sphere is open to creativity, in which pastors can certainly learn from their palliative colleagues.

5. Services of healing, of the kind practised by charismatics, and communal anointings of the sick (as at Lourdes, etc.) are meaningful and often an indication of a message of hope. People can pray without restraint for bodily and spiritual healing. A greater variety of such services can only do good. So there needs to be more than just a blessing of the dying.

6. But such communal services are not an alternative to the personal anointing of the sick. I share the view of Gisbert Greshake that a patient should be personally anointed when he or she is objectively and subjectively confronted with the possibility of dying in the first person.[9] Here my argument is both anthropological and theological. It is anthropological because people need a substantive rite of passage. And a rite of transition works only if it is ambiguous. It is theological because without equivocation such a ritual confronts the decisive question whether (looking back) I have died enough to be able to rise with Christ and whether (looking forward) I am ready with Christ to take the last step of surrendering my life. Thus according to Greshake the anointing of the sick is the sacrament of self-renewal in confrontation with death.

7. In the framework of the development of the ministries in the church it seems to me obvious that the priest should actively involve pastoral workers in the anointing of patients whom they have supported. This is not only a confirmation of their work, but also represents the continuity of care to the patient.

8. The blessing of the dying is also a good thing. This new rite is not put under pressure by a somewhat later anointing of the sick. I am not arguing for a return to Extreme Unction. The blessing of the dying is a liturgical act and thus to be performed primarily by a pastor. But if no hospital chaplain or pastoral worker is available, the situation challenges

every believer to take responsibility at the moment of dying of a fellow human being. In the present constellation of health care in Western Europe, with its high degree of technology, I do not directly see room for the viaticum as the very final liturgical gesture. I have already given the reasons for this. But there is no reason why it should not be a kind of 'solemn' communion, for example after the celebration of the sacrament of reconciliation. And if the sick person cannot receive communion, why should not his or her partner do so in their place? It could be a kind of completion of the sacrament of marriage.

Conclusion

The main concern of this article is the collaboration between carers, the family, volunteers, pastoral workers and hospital chaplains in supporting the terminally ill. In it sacraments are seen as a sealing of the indispensable contribution of each of these, while the work of each already has sacramental value. Because in this sphere too the situations all over the world are very different, this article is at the same time a plea for pluriformity. Such a difference is necessary if we are to be faithful to the essentials.

Translated by John Bowden

Notes

1. J.-L. Angué reports on his investigation in 'La mort et les funérailles en Europe', *La Maison-Dieu* 196, 1993.4, 19.

2. See e.g. K. Froggatt, 'Signposts on the Journey. The Place of Ritual in Spiritual Care', *International Journal of Palliative Nursing* 3, 1996, 42–6; S. Mayo, 'Symbol, Metaphor and Story. The Function of Group Art Therapy in Palliative Care', *Palliative Medicine* 10, 1996, 209–16.

3. Katrien Cornette investigated this in preparation for her doctoral thesis, *Spirituele zorg in palliatieve settings. Een bevraging van Vlaamse palliatieve zorgverleners*, Leuven 1997; there is a summary of the results of her research in 'For Whenever I Am Weak, I Am Strong. A National Survey into Spiritual Needs and Spiritual Growth among Palliative Caregivers', *International Journal of Palliative Nursing* 3, 1997, 6–13.

4. I have discussed these results in a wider context in 'Prier avec les mourants. Un nouveau rituel aux Pays-Bas', *La Maison-Dieu* 205, 1996/1, 91–106, and also in 'Naar een ontvouwing van het sacrament van de zieken? Over de zegening van een stervende', *Collationes* 27, 1997, 53–67.

5. There is a very good survey in A. van Eijk, 'Het pleidooi voor een ruimer sacramentsbegrip', in id. and H. Rikhof, *De lengte en de breedte, de oogte en de diepte. Peilingen in de theologie van de sacramenten*, Zoetermeer 1996, 106–31.

6. L. Boff, *Os Sacramentos da vida e a vida dos sacramentos*, Petropolis 1975.

7. F.-X. Durrwell, *L'Eucharistie, présence du Christ*, Paris 1971.

8. L.-M. Chauvet, *Les sacraments. Parole de Dieu au risque du corps*, Paris 1993, 81.

9. G. Greshake, 'Extreme Unction or Anointing of the Sick? A Plea for Discrimination', *Review for Religious* 45, 1986, 435–52.

Part III

Prayer Healing and Politics: The Quietism of the Healing Churches in Southern Africa

Matthew Schoffeleers

Summary

Christian missionaries by and large find it impossible to become so syncretistic as to share with their parishioners beliefs in witchcraft and other mystical forces causing sickness and assorted forms of misfortune. Consequently, (former) mission churches have been unable to develop an effective healing ministry. This is a disadvantage in so far as it forces 'mission Christians' to seek help elsewhere. But is also has its positive side, as it allows churches to engage in effective social criticism to a degree which seems beyond the healing churches. Hence, if a healing ministry is to be developed in the former missionary churches, it is recommended that measures be taken to safeguard their prophetic potential.

I. Introduction

Critics often make it appear as though all missionaries are heartless barbarians. True enough, there are those, mainly of the fundamentalist type, who – unhampered by excessive familiarity with the topic – routinely condemn African religion as immoral, superstitious, or even as the work of the devil. On the other hand, from the very beginning there also have been missionaries who not only did their utmost to acquire an often impressive knowledge of traditional religions, but who were also able to appreciate the many positive elements in those religions. Although such missionaries have formed a distinct minority, they have been influential beyond their number because of their publications, and because many of them also used to serve as instructors to newcomers to the mission field. One thinks particularly of people like Edwin Smith,

Placide Tempels and John V. Taylor – but there have been many more.[1] Their merit has been that they were among the first to demonstrate convincingly and in terms understandable to Westerners that African relFFigions contain ideas and values which may be a potential enrichment to Christianity. It is thanks to these studies that we can now speak of a flourishing African theology.

II. The aetiological system

Understandably, not all their colleagues felt able to agree with these innovators. To quite a few, the main obstacle was the African belief in witches, evil spirits and *nganga* or medicine persons – briefly, the entire aetiological and therapeutic system – which they found unacceptable.[2] In view of this it is interesting to note that people such as Smith, Tempels and Taylor discuss witchcraft and related beliefs only as side issues, as if they were of little more than secondary importance. Much the same can be said of African theology, which hardly ever discusses these topics. Indeed, African theology owes much of its attractiveness – particularly in the eyes of Westerners – to the fact that it carefully avoids such issues. But the price African theology has to pay for this is that it has been unable to develop a meaningful theology of sin and evil.[3] It therefore seems correct to conclude that as far as the mainstream churches are concerned, dialogue in the sense of a willingness to accept the reasonableness of the alternative viewpoint is possible only on condition that the African aetiological and therapeutical system is left out of consideration.

III. Healing churches and *ngangas*

That conclusion, however, does not apply to the leaders of the healing churches, also known as African Zionist churches.[4] One of the attractions of these churches is precisely that they share the kind of aetiological thinking of those who come to them for help, but at the same time they have developed diagnostic and therapeutic techniques of their own which, in their eyes and those of their clients, are 'safer' because they are considered less tainted with witchcraft. The Workshop on Christian Independency at the Harare Conference of the International Association for Mission Studies (IAMS) issued a report which states that:

> Generally speaking it is possible to effect truly genuine and lasting healing within the African context only if this fundamental cause of evil [i.e. witchcraft] is taken very seriously and is dealt with adequately.

Most mission churches and some African Independent Churches simply reject, repudiate and then ignore witchcraft, forcing people to live schizophrenically in two different worlds. It must be stated that this constitutes an entirely deficient response to witchcraft. Witchcraft, sorcery and wizardry might well be useful as a paradigm of the Devil, a fruitful point of contact for the development of a meaningful doctrine of sin and evil.[5] Just how 'schizophrenic' the life of mission Christians is I am unable to say, but judging from studies by Murphree, Kuper, and others, one would be inclined to think that most people do not find it difficult to combine Christianity with traditional religion.[6] Whatever the truth, it is important to note that the established churches apparently prefer to leave that part of their pastoral task which concerns the evil perpetrated by witches and malevolent spirits to the *ngangas* and the healing prophets, rather than engage in it themselves. It is the price they are prepared to pay for keeping themselves free of syncretism (International Organization for Mission Studies, Christian Mission and Human Transformation, *Mission Studies* 2, no. 1, 1985).

IV. Milingo's healing ministry

Yet from the early 1960s onwards, when the liberation struggle in Africa reached its zenith and mission churches were busy Africanizing their cadres, voices were being raised to plead for a healing ministry in the mainstream churches.[7] One of the best known representatives of this movement is undoubtedly Emmanuel Milingo, the former Catholic Archbishop of Lusaka.[8] The facts about this man are generally known. Having begun his healing ministry in 1973, he was forced in July 1983 to offer his resignation as Archbishop after a protracted conflict with his own clergy, his fellow bishops, and the Vatican. Exiled to Rome, where he was offered a post in the papal commission for the pastorate among migrants and tourists, he was nevertheless allowed, although not whole-heartedly – to continue his healing ministry on a more or less regular basis. It is not altogether clear what the Vatican holds against him, since a formal charge has never been made public, but Mona MacMillan, who edited and published a selection from Milingo's writings, suggests in her introduction that among other things Rome was afraid of a schism.[9] Fear was also expressed that the public might in the end regard Milingo as one of the many *ngangas*, 'perhaps more powerful and certainly cheaper than the rest'. That he saw himself as replacing the traditional *ngangas* is clear from what he wrote in a private letter: 'There are a thousand and one

African doctors who claim to have mysterious powers. They charge a lot of money and they cannot stand that I have the people they would have had.'[10]

Aylward Shorter, missionary, anthropologist and prolific writer on matters concerning African Christianity, further accuses Milingo of imposing 'a fundamentalist demonological theory on African spirit mediumship, which has more in common with the *Malleus Maleficarum* of fifteenth-century Europe than with any tradition found in Africa'.[11] It is to be hoped that Shorter does not really mean it when he says that Milingo's ideas have little to do with African religious tradition, for it is clear that those very ideas are shared by literally thousands of prophet healers in the Independent Churches, of whom there can be no doubt that they stand fully in the African tradition.

The charge against Milingo is therefore fundamentally that his ministry is a threat to Christian orthodoxy and ecclesiastical unity. The first charge does not seem that serious, since he is allowed to continue his healing ministry outside Africa. The real charge is likely to be the second. The Vatican was probably afraid that Milingo's enormous success might lead to similar movements elsewhere in Africa and possibly to serious schisms.[12] By way of conclusion we may therefore note that the dialogue between Western-style Christianity and traditional religion seems to have reached its critical point in the likes of Milingo, and once again it is clear that the dialogue flounders on the subject of African aetiology.

V. Social criticism

One might regard what happened to Milingo as yet another instance of Vatican meddlesomeness and leave it at that. The point, however, is that most healing ministries raise a problem of a different kind, which is that they are, socially speaking, very conservative. Time and again one notices that churches and movements which are heavily involved in ritual healing seem to lose their capability for engaging in social criticism and activism. By that phrase I am referring to the capability of the church to protest openly by word and deed against oppressive structures and institutions. Experts are unanimous in stating that healing churches avoid oppositional political commitment.[13] Kaja Finkler, an anthropologist who carried out research among a popular Christian healing movement in Mexico, found this conservative attitude even in movements which are critical of the social structures to which they are subject. According to Finkler, ritual healing illustrates in the clearest possible way the contradiction in the healing process, which is directed at the well-being of the individual, but which at the same time supports the social structure directly or indirectly responsible for his or her illness.[14] Her conclusion is therefore that to change social structures or to effect a significant social transformation one needs personalities which stand outside healing movements, a thesis which seemed convincingly illustrated by the situation in South Africa, where ecclesiastical protest against apartheid was by and large a matter for churches without a strong healing tradition.

VI. Conclusion

Despite these reservations about religious healing I would plead for the recognition of a healing ministry in the African Christian communities. My reason for saying so is that religious healing undeniably represents a therapeutic potential which other forms of healing do not possess. Having said this, I can think of two ways of saving the healing ministry.

1. The mainline churches could acknowledge the value of the healing pastorate, but prefer to leave it in the hands of traditional healers and healing prophets. This is not as fantastic as it sounds, for it is precisely this which happens nowadays from one end of sub-Saharan Africa to the other. It would imply, however, that the mainstream churches would have to recognize those healers and prophets and co-operate with them. This would leave those churches themselves available for the struggle against social injustice, which is what we have been seeing in South Africa at the height of apartheid.

2. A second possibility would be to have the mainstream churches organize a dual ministry, consisting of the present ministry of word and sacrament, alongside a ministry of healing, in which the laity would be involved as well. The former would take care of issues concerning social justice, while the second would take care of the suffering individual. The advantage in this case would be that the church would be in a position – at least in theory – to discourage and reduce syncretism.

Bibliography

H. Adam and K. Moodley, *South Africa Without Apartheid: Dismantling Racial Domination*, Los Angeles/London 1986.

IAMS, *Christian Mission and Human Transformation*, Mission Studies 2, no. 1, 1985.

K. Finkler, 'The Social Consequence of Wellness: A View of Healing Outcomes from Micro and Macro Perspectives', *International Journal of Health Services* 16, 1986, 627–42.

L. Kretschmar, *The Voice of Black Theology in Southern Africa*, Johannesburg 1986.

A. Kuper, 'The Magician and the Missionary', in *The Liberal Dilemma in South Africa*, ed. P. L. van den Berghe, London 1979, 1–62.

L. Lagerwerf, 'Witchcraft, Sorcery and Spirit Possession: Pastoral Responses in Africa', *Exchange* 14, no. 41, 1985, 1–62.

E. Milingo, *The World in Between: Christian Healing and the Struggle for Spiritual Survival*, New York 1984.

M. W. Murphree, *Christianity and the Shona*, London 1979.

M. Schoffeleers, 'Black Theology and African Theology in Southern Africa: An Old Controversy Re-examined', *Journal of Religion in Africa* 18, no. 2, 1988, 99–124.

M. Schoffeleers, 'Ritual Healing and Political Acquiescence. The Case of the Zionist Churches in South Africa', *Africa*, Vol. 61, 1991, no. 1, 1–25.

A. Shorter, *Jesus and the Witchdoctor: An Approach to Healing and Wholeness*, New York 1985.

E. W. Smith (ed.), *African Ideas of God*, London 1960.

B. Sundkler, *Bantu Prophets in South Africa*, London 1961.

J. V. Taylor, *The Primal Vision*, London 1963.

P. Tempels, *La Philosophie Bantoue*, Elisabethville 1945.

Notes

1. Smith 1960; Tempels 1945; Taylor 1963.
2. Bucher 1980; Hammond Tooke 1986.
3. Schoffeleers 1988.
4. Sundkler 1961.
5. IAMS 1985.
6. Murphree 1969, 150–1; Kuper 1979, 77–96.
7. See among others Lagerwerf 1985, which contains a chronological survey of colloquia and documents.
8. For a summary of Milingo's ideas, see Milingo 1984.
9. Mona MacMillan, Introduction to Milingo 1984.
10. Milingo 1984, 5.
11. Shorter 1985, 190.
12. See Shorter 1985, 191, for a Tanzanian case of a Catholic priest-healer.
13. Kretschmar, 1986, 52–5; Adam and Moodley, 1986, 201–2.
14. Finkler 1986, 627–42.

New Church Practices in Healing. Their Importance in Asian High Cultures: India

Eliza Kuppozhackel

The health care system in India today is at the cross roads. Over-reliance on high technology and the craze for super-specialization, together with the increasing cost of health care, make a health service an impossible dream for the teeming millions of India. The institutionalized approach which has been mainly following the allopathic system with its focus on a curative and preventive approach is being challenged by the emerging new trends which focus on a holistic and integrated approach in health promotion. These modes emphasize the total well-being of the person rather than dealing with the symptoms of illness; they use low-cost traditional systems of medicine, non-drug therapies and energy-balancing techniques. The church in India, in its attempt to follow Jesus' healing ministry, is being caught up in the web of the modern consumerist medical approach. There is a need to reframe its approach and opt for total health and holistic healing for the welfare of the people of the country.

Health care in the pre- and post-independence period

The church in India made a great contribution in the field of health care, together with that of education. Health care of ordinary people became one of the main concerns of all missionary groups right from the sixteenth century. This was all the more urgent, since large sections of poor people had absolutely no opportunity to get the services of physicians, who belonged to the upper castes. The poor had recourse only to ritualistic practices, incantations and black magic. Allopathy, which came with trade and colonization, was promoted in India by the British. In the post-independence period, the nation adopted allopathy as the national system of medicine, to the neglect of all other systems. The church too accepted Western allopathic medicine, finding it more systematic and empirical and consequently more effective and confidence-building.

Medical missions flourished in India with the decree *Constans Ac Sedula*, granting permission to religious to practise obstetrics and surgery (1936). Medical educational institutions like the Christian Medical College at Vellore, Christian Medical College at Ludhiana and St John's Medical College at Bangalore developed along with several nursing schools and para-medical training centres attached to large hospitals. The poor had health facilities made available through the church's many health-care institutions, which were mainly in the rural and semi-urban areas. These institutions were highly developed, effective and affordable until extreme sophistication began to set in.

A new crisis in health care

Gradually the health care system in India developed all the specialization and sophistication that evolved in the West, without asking the question whether India could afford it or needed it. Mega-technologies and super-specialization, along with high cost of medicine, made health care a rare commodity for the vast majority. Lack of responsibility for their own health made people over-dependent on medicine, doctors and hospitals. Medical drugs were easily available over the counter even without proper prescription. 'Banned and bannable drugs',[1] along with spurious products, filled the market. Curative treatment of the body without tackling the psycho-spiritual and social factors underlying the ailment was the main approach. One could say that the very health care system itself became sick.

The prevalent medical technology is marked by an analytical approach which came with the modern Western medical education: whatever is measurable and objective through the Western scientific model became the norm of medical practice. There is a subject–object dichotomy where the *subject*, the knower, knows the *object* and masters it. The doctor claims to know everything and the patient is a passive receiver. Domination or subjugation is the process even in the relationship and all related transactions. Everything is separated from everything else. Hence the dominant exploit natural resources for their well-being at the cost of those less powerful.

The church-related hospitals and health institutions began to struggle for survival. They had to pay high salaries to maintain doctors. There is no justice in this payment, as it widens the gap between the rich and poor. In Christian hospitals too there is a big difference between the salary of the doctors and that of the lower-grade employees. Many doctors also demand payment through illegal channels. In Kerala many hospitals are forced to adjust these amounts from the salary of the religious sisters or the other staff working there. The craze for specialists and famous doctors who can attract patients to a hospital has naturally led to high-level competition among private hospitals. This is most evident in church-related health institutions. In such a competitive atmosphere even Christian institutions appear to be business concerns run on the profit motive. They become increasingly inaccessible to the poor. The patients have to spend a lot of money on expensive tests even before any treatment starts. A major sickness in the family makes them financially bankrupt. Health, which should be maintained through proper diet and nutrition, is affected by their increased poverty. They become chronically ill instead of moving higher on the scale of health and well-being.

Emerging new trends

Conscientious people started questioning the state of affairs in the field of health and development. As a result, the traditional Indian systems of healing that survived the onslaught of Western medicine attracted attention. People began to accept several non-drug therapies in an effort to promote health and wholeness. Ayruveda, Sidha, Unani, Yoga, herbal medicine, tribal medicine, Pranic healing, Reiki, naturopathy, oriental medicine, counselling, pastoral care, etc. found their way into the integrated approach to health and as a means of low-cost and self-help techniques. Some of the hospitals and community health centres introduced these methods along with modern medicine. 'Unlike modern systems of health care which are reductionist and based on Newtonian logic, traditional health care is holistic and based on non-exploitative relations between man and nature.'[2] The holistic health movement that started emerging in the West also influenced the Indian attempt at a redefinition of health. There is today a general reawakening in people's approach to health and sickness.

A return to traditional systems: restoring harmony and balance

The whole philosophy behind this reawakening is again nothing drastically new; it is only a return to our age-old traditions and cultural heritage. The non-drug therapies believe in the self-regulatory mechanism of the body and its power to heal itself from within. Medicine is seen as an aid to activate the healing potential of the body and not an attack on it. Instead of putting emphasis on surgery and the removal of unhealthy organs, these forms of therapy see illness as an imbalance in the system and healing as restoring the balance. It is the person who is treated and not the symptoms of his ailment. Contrary to the analytical approach, it is an ontological approach that is the approach of the Vedas and the Upanishads of India (1200–500 BC). Knowledge is a way of being and not geared to subjugation and domination; it assumes self-responsibility for health and healthy behaviour. It is not a rational but an intuitive approach, in which one becomes aware of the interconnectedness of everything at a deep level. It is not based on subject–object polarity, but on being in communion with one's core and with the cosmic reality. There is unity and relationality in all things. Knowledge leads to self-transformation. Healing is a personal response to live according to the rhythm of reality.

According to the Indian understanding, each human being is composed of five sheaths of reality which are called *kōsa* in Sanskrit.[3] The existential harmony in the human being is sustained by the harmonic balance of these sheaths. The outer sheath is known as *annamaya kōsa* (physical body) and is sustained by the food (matter) we eat. The second sheath consists of *prānamaya kōsa* (vital life force), which is gained by exposing oneself to the energy sources such as air, sunlight and earth. *Mañomaya kōsa* is made up of the emotional element in the human being, while *vigjānamaya kōsa* is the creation of acquired knowledge. The core of human existence is the *ānandamaya kōsa*, the divine bliss, which is the abode of the Supreme; this is the core-potential which radiates light on the other four sheaths and integrates the person. Each superior sheath keeps the inferior sheath in touch with the centre of our being, which is *ānandamaya kōsa*. In this view human health is the harmony of all these levels of existence: physical, vital, emotional, rational and spiritual. Distortion of the unity and integration of these layers is known as illness. Hence healing has to be addressed to the appropriate levels of existence from where disharmony begins.

All material bodies, according to the Sankhya and Vedanta, have evolved from the interaction between *prakrti*, the dynamic and material principle, and *purusha*, the spirit of universal consciousness. All that is present in the cosmos has its existence in the person too. According to the theory of *Pancha-bhuta*, the physical body (*annamaya kosa*) of the person and the physical nature of the cosmos are both made of five elements: earth, water, fire, wind and etheric space. If any of these elements subdues or dominates the other an imbalance occurs, which is the cause of ailments. This principle is implied in the treatment modalities of acupuncture, acupressure and Sujok. The treatment called naturopathy also makes use of diet, exercise, earth, water and sunlight to restore wholeness. Food is the real medicine: controlled diet evokes vital energies. Through fasting the body absorbs the assimilative energy of the etheric space. Healing in the sense of the Atharva Veda is to regain the lost interconnectedness through the chanting of certain sacred verses and the performance of sacred rites. Ayurveda, an Indian system of medicine, also holds this idea when it speaks of *dosha* (imbalance) of the three humours, *vātha* (wind), *pitha* (bile) and *kapha* (secretions) in the body as the basis of all physical maladies.[4] The human person is considered as part of the cosmic existence because the person is a microcosm. The cosmic symphony is expressed not only in the universe but also in the human body. A healthy human body vibrates harmoniously according to its own nature. When this harmony is distorted, the result is imbalance and sickness. This musical harmony is restored through body massage using oil, herbal medicine, finger pressure and different types of heat therapy. Yogic *āsana* and *prānayama* also aid in harmonizing and balancing the body-rhythm and vibrations.

Beyond empirical analysis

The Indian systems of healing and restoring harmony cannot be adequately measured by analytical tools because the Indian methods transcend the boundaries of empirical science. In health and healing there are always subjective and objective elements. For example, the body temperature can be measured by a thermometer, but the subjective experience of feverishness cannot be measured. An experienced practitioner of Eastern medicine can identify and sense it through feeling the body vibration as well as the energy field (aura) surrounding the body. Let us consider the practice of Pranic healing, for example. In Pranic healing a person is understood as consisting of a 'subtle body' (*sūkhsma sarira*) besides his or her gross physical body (*sthūla sarira*). *Prāna* (vital force) keeps the body alive and active by its circulation through the body. There are specific energy centres called '*chakras*' which absorb vital energy directly from the atmosphere and distribute it to different parts of the body. A Pranic healer with his/her trained hand can diagnose whether the enegies are flowing harmoniously. While treating, the healer opens himself/herself to the divine cosmic energy and becomes a channel to re-establish the energy balance that was lost in the person.

Wholeness as holiness

Harmony, balance, integration, unity and mutual interrelation of all things and events characterize the Indian approach to health, healing and wholeness. Everything is part of the whole, and there is a basic flow and rhythm that maintains this unity and oneness. Ultimate reality is expressed and experienced in different manifestations of the Cosmic Whole. In this sense health and spirituality are one and the same. Both are directed to wholeness, fullness of life, purity and integration. Wholeness is holiness.

Jesus Christ came to heal and restore the lost harmony and balance. Healing and wholeness was the establishment of the kingdom. Judaism insisted on the Law, which is an outward observance that neglects the human spirit. Though Jesus healed the body, he insisted on the spirit of the human person. Jesus always asked those who approached him for healing what they wanted. Thus he involved the seeker in his/her healing process, eliciting faith and self-responsibility. Healing the malady always led to a total transformation in the person. The blind man was able to see, but his inner eyes were opened to see Jesus as the messiah.

The incarnation of the Logos and the resurrection of Christ can be seen as the divine affirmation of our bodily existence. God came to us through the body, and we reach God through the body. Body is the primary place of encountering the divine; body is the primal sacrament, the temple of the divine Spirit. Our body is a grace and a responsibility. Caring for a healthy body is our response to the incarnational self-giving of God in Christ. However, body is not just a biological reality; it is the totality of the self-expression of the human. Hence we believe in the 'resurrection of the body'. Health is a holistic experience that demands concern for bodily well-being, psychic harmony and spiritual integration. Ultimately our caring for health is our participation in the healing work of the divine Spirit that makes everything new and restores all things in the Risen Christ until the moment when 'God will be all in all'.

The church's healing mission stems from the mission of Jesus and his command 'Go, preach and heal'. The basic attitude of the church to the sick has to be that of loving-kindness and caring with compassion. When health care became extremely sophisticated, the soul-searching questions and analysis by several groups within the church discovered alternative approaches to health care with emphasis on a holistic and integrated approach. The Ayushya centre for healing and integration at Changanacherry, Kerala; Holy Family Hospital, Patna; Bihar, and several others can be cited as examples. The Catholic Hospital Association of India and Christian Medical Association of India, extended their support to the new approach to health care. Health education today is assuring a greater role in bringing back health consciousness to its innate quality of well-being through a healthy life-style, in the light of the Indian view on integration with nature's rhythm.

Conclusion

The church took the initiative at a time when health care was needed through hospitals. Today's consciousness is directed at a new approach in health care. Changes have started with small committed groups, but the official church has yet to clarify its stand. Its challenge today is to be a credible witness to the sublime values of the Indian and the Christian heritage of healing ministry.

Notes

1. See *Banned and Bannable Drugs* (brought out in the public interest by the Voluntary Health Association of India), first published 1986; Third Revised Edition, May 1989.
2. Kali Chattergee, 'In Search of an Alternative', in Alok Mukhopadhyay (ed.), *State of India's Health*, Delhi 1992, 163.
3. See Haridas Bhattacharyya (ed.), *The Cultural Heritage of India*, Vol. III, Calcutta 1953, 589.
4. See Priyadaranjan Ray and S. N. Sen (eds.), *The Cultural Heritage of India*, Vol. VI, 164–5.

Illness and Healing in the Uamsho (Revival) Movement in Tanzania

Anneth Munga

Introduction

Within any human society, the question of healing is a crucial one. In Africa, where medical services rarely counterbalance the prevalence of illnesses and maladies that afflict people, the search for cure is an important part of the struggle for survival. Indeed, to discuss the topic of healing in Africa from a theological perspective is to deal with an existential concern of most Africans. In this article, I explore how healing is practised and understood in the revival groups that operate within the Evangelical Lutheran Church in Tanzania. After an introduction to the revival movement in Tanzania, I describe the revivalists' understanding of the cause of sickness. I then consider the process of healing itself, and present the arguments used by revivalists to legitimize healing. Afterwards, I discuss the relationship of the revivalists' idea of healing to the practice of traditional healers and in the conclusion I offer some additional comments. My focus is on physical illness and physical healing.

The Swahili term for revival is *Uamsho*,[1] and the revival movement in Tanzania is to be referred to as the *Uamsho* movement. The adherents of the *Uamsho* movement are *wanauamsho* (singular – *mwanauamsho*).

A presentation of the *Uamsho* movement in Tanzania[2]

The *Uamsho* movement is part of the East African Revival Movement that began in the 1920s. It covers most parts of Kenya, Uganda, Tanzania, Rwanda, Burundi, eastern Zaire and the southern areas of Sudan. The *Uamsho* movement consists of local groups within the

Protestant churches and it functions under the leadership of lay men and women, *wanauamsho*.[3] The gathering of a local group is called *faragha* or fellowship, and the participants are those who regard themselves as already saved, although others are allowed to attend as well.[4] The activities during *faragha* are: singing songs and choruses, prayer, welcoming newcomers, confession of sin, bearing testimonies, reading the Bible, preaching, commenting on the sermon, and collecting offerings. In their proclamation, *wanauamsho* mainly emphasize salvation and living in holiness. Elements not always included in *faragha* are speaking in tongues, praying for sick people and exorcism. Apart from *faragha* there are two other forms of meetings: spiritual conventions and seminars. Because of their in-church character, these groups comply with the administration of sacraments as practised in the respective congregations. They also lack any form of hierarchy, although some *wanauamsho* have become well-known preachers throughout Tanzania. *Uamsho* groups function ecumenically, and *wanauamsho* cooperate regardless of their differences in terms of social status, tribal identity, nationality and race.

The understanding of sickness in *Uamsho*

Regardless of scientifically verifiable factors, Satan is believed by *wanauamsho* to be part of the explanation behind maladies that afflict human beings. A distinct feature in the understanding of the existence of sickness among *wanauamsho* is the emphasis on the existence and activity of demons.[5]

Regarding demon possession, *wanauamsho* can be grouped into two main wings. First, there is the extreme wing with a pan-demonic view. Those who hold this view believe that every hardship, including sickness, is caused by demons. One may be possessed by demons through contact with relatives or friends who have demons. The second wing of *wanauamsho* have a moderate perception of demons in the sense that they regard demons as a possible but not necessary cause of sickness.

While Satan is seen as the intrinsic source of illness, the absence of God's protection is also understood as a possible cause of sickness. It means that the involvement of God in the existence of sickness is secondary and occurs by God permitting its occurrence. Therefore sickness is explained both as a reality in itself and as the absence of something good.

First, *wanauamsho* believe that God can permit sickness as a punishment for sin. The holiness and sovereignty of God does not only guarantee his ability to conquer Satan; these attributes also justify God's vengeance upon the sinner. God has both the ability and right to punish offenders just as he did with the Israelites, as shown in the Old Testament. However, the view of a punishing God can also be explained by the Tanzanian cultural parameters according to which the role of the father incorporates the right and duty to discipline his children.

Secondly, *wanauamsho* believe that God can permit sickness for a good purpose. Here, *wanauamsho* use the principle of double effect. Sickness may help a person to attain the highest good, which is salvation now and eternal life in heaven in the life hereafter.

The process of healing

Jesus Christ is understood by *wanauamsho* as the ultimate healer. Therefore, *wanauamsho* emphasize that the salvific work of Jesus Christ includes deliverance of the human being from the bondage of Satan. An important efficacy of the death of Jesus Christ on the cross is liberation from the 'powers of darkness'. The blood of Jesus Christ is understood to be significant for the healing of a sick person.

There are two key terms which *wanauamsho* use in legitimizing the exercise of the gift of healing: ability (*uwezo*) and authority (*mamlaka*). Apart from acting as the communicator between God and human beings, the Holy Spirit gives the saved person the ability to exercise spiritual gifts such as exorcism and healing. The fact that people are not only being delivered from sickness and demons but also make the decision to follow Jesus proves the legitimacy of healing as one among other spiritual gifts. If the exercise of a spiritual gift brings about the conversion of an unconverted person, this is in itself a legitimization of that gift.

Authority derives from Jesus Christ, with whom the saved ones are exalted and through whom they reign as kings. *Uamsho* bases its perception of 'Jesus as the ultimate healer' on the New Testament accounts of exorcisms and healing. If Jesus was able to heal sick people and cast out demons during his stay on earth two thousand years ago, there is no reason why this should not be possible today. Those who are saved are heirs together with Christ and share with him the same spirit of God. Therefore, the saved ones have the authority to use the name of Jesus when using the gift of healing. The status of heir and the sharing of God's spirit are matters of 'all sharing everything', because all those who are saved are on an equal level with Christ, with whom they share his sonship and therefore his inheritance rights.

There are *wanauamsho* who believe that not all saved ones possess all gifts. On the basis of that view, not every saved person has the particular gift of healing. However, other *wanauamsho* argue that it is wrong to excuse oneself from participating in healing. Being delivered from Satan and the powers of darkness is a subjective experience, but it is also received as an object by the saved person. The moment a person is saved, he or she automatically acquires the ability to combat the power of Satan by receiving ability and authority. With the ability of the Holy Spirit given to a person who receives Jesus as the saviour of his life and with the authority which all saved ones have in Christ, their brother and co-heir, any genuinely saved person should be able to carry out tasks such a expelling demons.

There are two ways in which *wanauamsho* exercise healing. One alternative is to pray for healing in a calm manner during, for instance, a spiritual convention. The *mwanauamsho* who is preaching in that gathering might claim that he or she has been told by the Holy Spirit about a specific person with a specific health problem. The preacher then prays for this unidentified person, after which the convention continues as planned. The following day, the preacher informs the convention participants that he or she has been told by the Holy Spirit that the person prayed for the day before is present and has been partially or fully healed. Without knowing who this person is, he or she is asked to come forward and testify about that healing. Afterwards, the participants in the meeting sing and the preacher says a prayer of praise to God.

The second way of practising healing is exorcism, which is more dramatic than the former way. Exorcism is carried out either during an *Uamsho* gathering or as a separate session. If exorcism takes place as a continuation of a spiritual convention, sick people who are absent from that gathering can be represented by family members who have attended. In other words, it is believed that deliverance from demons can take place indirectly.

Normally, the procedure of exorcism has five phases:[6]

(i) *The preparatory phase*: sometimes it is expected in advance that exorcism will be carried out. A few *wanauamsho* prepare themselves for that task through individual meditation, prayer and fasting.

(ii) *Praise and repentance*: this is the first part of the exorcism prayer itself. Repeatedly and with loud voices, those who are to carry out exorcism may pray as follows: 'In the name of Jesus Christ of Nazareth Our God we glorify you . . . You are the only one, our God, the only one. There is no one else, God, like you . . . forgive us for we have sinned, sinned before you, have mercy, have mercy God . . .'

(iii) *The diagnostic phase*: this consists in a 'dispute' between the demons and the exorcists (*wanauamsho*). The demons are believed to express themselves through their host:

Exorcist	Demons
'Who are you?'	'And who are you?'
'We are the servant of the Lord Jesus.'	'And we are many.'
'How many are you?'	'Two.'
'How long have you been in this person?'	'For three years.'
'But now Jesus Christ of Nazareth wants you to leave this person whom you have tortured for all this time.'	'We are not leaving.'
'In the name of Jesus Christ we command you, leave this person.'	'We are not leaving, where are we to go then?'
'Return to the one who sent you, etc.'	

(iv) *The therapeutic phase*: during this phase a prayer is said in order to expel the demons from their host. The phrases 'in the name of Jesus and the blood of Jesus' are repeated until the host is believed to have been freed. By touching, exorcism is directed to those parts of the body which the demons are believed to inhabit.

(v) *The prophylactic phase*: during this phase, hands are laid upon house walls and utensils used by the formerly demon-possessed person.

The relationship between the idea of healing in the *Uamsho* movement and the practices of traditional healers

There are scholars who concede that in sub-Saharan Africa there is a christological paradigm according to which the role of Jesus Christ is conceived in analogy with that of the African traditional healer, in Swahili known as *mganga*.[7] Among *wanauamsho*, there is an outspoken resentment at traditional healers. However there is a substantial difference between the view of *wanauamsho* and that of the early Western missionaries with regard to traditional healers. The missionaries dismissed the African traditional religious practices, including the practices of traditional healers, regarding them as superstition and paganism. However, *wanauamsho* take the practices of traditional healers seriously. Therefore, during exorcism in *Uamsho* groups, those amulets which the sick people have previously obtained from traditional healers so as to obtain protection from evil powers are treated by *wanauamsho* as highly potential carriers of demons. In order to destroy the suspected demons, the amulets are burnt up. The paradox is this: the very amulets that are supposed to function *prophylactically* when provided by traditional healers become objects of *therapeutic* activity when *wanauamsho* exercise the gift of healing. For *wanauamsho*, amulets do not *prevent* sickness; rather they *cause* sickness. Yet, as in the case of *wanauamsho*, the traditional healers use the diagnostic, therapeutic and prophylactic stages when carrying out their activities.

One may therefore observe that the content of the notion of Jesus as the ultimate healer among *wanauamsho* is, to a significant extent, influenced by the practices of traditional healers. Paradoxically, though, *wanauamsho* emphasize the theme of Jesus as the ultimate healer because of their claim on *discontinuity* between the Christian faith and the practices of traditional healers. The relationship between the idea of healing in the *Uamsho* movement and the practices of traditional healers is antagonistic, yet the former is clearly influenced by the latter.

Conclusion

The focus on healing among *wanauamsho* stems from a genuine concern among people within as well as outside the *Uamsho* movement. *wanauamsho* are addressing an existential issue that is deeply rooted in the lives of Africans. Basing themselves on the New Testament accounts of healing and on the idea that a person acquires ability and authority at the moment of conversion, *wanauamsho* legitimize the exercise of healing. In spite of the discontinuity between the notion of Jesus as the ultimate healer among *wanauamsho* and the practices of traditional healers, *wanauamsho* are clearly influenced by the latter. Thus, *Uamsho's* idea of healing differs both from the Western missionaries' rejection of traditional healers and from the appreciation of the role of traditional healers as expressed within many African independent churches.

I would finally like to offer a few comments.

First, I have shown above that *wanauamsho* explain the fact that God allows sickness by appealing to the principle of double effect. I have also shown that such a perception of God can result from the influence of the ideas about the father's role in the Tanzanian family structure. Yet most Christians today find it hard to reconcile the image of a God who 'permits' suffering such as sickness with that of a benevolent and caring God. Moreover, it is no longer possible consistently to deny the link between the widespread poverty and insufficient medical services in most African countries on the one hand, and the prevailing unjust economic order that benefits less than a quarter of the world's population on the other. It is regrettable, I feel, that *wanauamsho*, who otherwise condemn sin very bluntly, do not address the sinful global systems that continue to reduce the chances for many Africans to maintain good health.

Secondly, with regard to sickness and healing, one misses the experience of those who have the most significant role in taking care of the sick, namely the women. It is the women who tirelessly combine numerous daily activities with the tasks of nurturing and nursing the sick in their homes or at hospitals. Somehow, they succeed in working out the impossible combination of time-consuming domestic duties in supporting their large families with the role of attending practically as well as emotionally to their sick relatives, neighbours and friends. Although women within the *Uamsho* movement participate on the same basis as men in the activity of proclamation, one does not find attributes such as self-dedication, patience and compassion reflected when *wanauamsho* describe God's involvement in the situation of the sick. Such 'motherly' prerogatives would offer a healthy balance to *wanauamsho's* view of God as a strict, punishing father.

Thirdly, the extreme stance of those *wanauamsho* who hold a pandemonic view has caused pastoral problems in some congregations within the Evangelical Lutheran Church of Tanzania. Also, while the idea that every saved person possesses ability and authority to use the name of Jesus against the powers of darkness has the potentiality of promoting an egalitarian ecclesiology, the question of who should expel demons has led to heated controversies among clergy as well as church members. In my view, such problems need to be dealt with not only at the pastoral level; they should also be included in the academic theological debate.

All in all, *wanauamsho* address a basic life-question among most people in Africa. By its clear focus on the question of sickness and healing, the *Uamsho* movement makes an important contribution both to African Christianity and to the theological reflection in Africa.

Notes

1. Swahili, a blend of Bantu and Arabic languages, is the national language of Tanzania and is spoken in other East African countries as well.

2. For a comprehensive systematic exploration of the *Uamsho* movement and its theology, see Anneth Nyagawa Munga, *Uamsho: A Theological Study of the Proclamation of the Revival Movement within the Evangelical Lutheran Church in Tanzania*, Studia Theologica Lundensia 54, Lund 1998.

3. Cf. Wilson Niwagila, *From the Catacomb to a Self-Governing Church: A Case Study of the African Initiative and the Participation of the Foreign Missions in the Mission History of the North-Western Diocese of the Evangelical Lutheran Church in Tanzania, 1890–1965,* Hamburg 1988, 248.

4. Cf. Bengt Sundkler, *Bare Bukoba: Church and Community in Tanzania,* London 123, 125.

5. *Wanauamsho* describe demons as harmful spirits which behave anthropomorphically.

6. With minor modifications, I have presented this procedure of exorcism in Munga, *Uamsho,* 287–8.

7. See Matthew Schoffeleers, 'Folk Christology: The Dialectics of the Nganga Paradigm', *Journal of Religion in Africa* 19, no. 2, 1989, 158. According to Schoffeleers, the *nganga* paradigm is used at the level of 'talk theology' in sub-Saharan Africa, while the 'intellectual elite' have never taken it seriously.

Contributors

PAUL J. PHILIBERT is Director of the Institute for Church Life at the University of Notre Dame. He is a Dominican priest. His writings focus on moral and religious development and on the interpretation of religious research.

Address: Institute for Church Life, University of Notre Dame, 1201 Hesburgh Library, Notre Dame, Indiana 46556, USA.

ERIC DE ROSNY was born in Fontainebleau in 1930 and became a Jesuit in 1947. He arrived in Douala, Cameroon in 1957, where he taught; he was appointed chaplain at the University of Yaoundé in 1965. Between 1970 and 1975 he continued his research on traditional medicine in South Cameroon and between 1975 to 1982 he was Director of the African Institute for Economic and Social Development at Abidjan, Ivory Coast. From 1984 to 1990 he was Jesuit Provincial for West Africa; he is now Director of the Spiritual Centre for Encounter at Douala, Cameroon. His books include *Healers in The Night*, Maryknoll 1985; *L'Afrique des guérisons*, Paris 1994; and *La nuit, les yeux ouverts*, Paris 1996. He has written around forty articles.

Address: Centre de Rencontre, PB 633, Douala, Cameroon.

MICHAEL NÜCHTERN was born in 1949, and is an ordained pastor. He is head of theology at the Protestant Centre for Ideological Questions in Berlin, and previously was Director of the Evangelische Akademie of Baden in Karlsruhe/Bad Herranalb. His most recent books are *Medizin, Magie, Moral, Über Therapie und Weltanschauung*, Mainz and Stuttgart 1995; *Kirche und Konkurrenz*, Stuttgart 1997.

Address: Evangelische Zentralstelle für Weltanschauungsfragen Berlin, Auguststrasse 80, D 10117 Berlin, Germany.

LARS THIELMANN was born in 1966 and studied Catholic theology at the Ruhr University, Bochum and medicine at Cologne University. Since October 1997 he has been a graduate member of the Centre for Ethics in the Sciences at the University of Tübingen. He is working on the ethical aspects of the allocation of resources in the health sector.

Address: Zentrum für Ethik in den Wissenschaften, Keplerstrasse 17, D 72074 Tübingen, Germany.

JEAN DELUMEAU was born in Nantes in 1923; he graduated in history and has a doctorate in letters. Until his retirement in 1994 he taught at the University of Rennes II, the Panthéon Sorbonne and then at the Collège de France. He is a member of the Institut. His main works are *Vie économique et sociale de Rome dans le second moitié du XVIe Siècle,* Paris 1957–9; *Naissance et affirmation de la Réforme,* Paris 1965; *La Civilisation de la Renaissance,* Paris 1967, *Le Catholicisme entre Luther et Voltaire,* Paris 1971; *Le Christianisme va-t-il mourir?,* Paris 1977; *Une histoire du Paradis* (2 vols), Paris 1992, 1995; *Les Religions et les Hommes,* Paris 1997.

Address: 29, rue des Lauriers, 35510 Cesson-Sevigne, France.

JEAN-CLAUDE LARCHET was born in 1949 at Badonviller, France. A patrologist and Orthodox theologian, he has a doctorate in theology from the University of Strasbourg and a doctorate in philosophy. His works include: *Théologie de la maladie,* Paris ²1994; *Therapeutique des maladies mentales. L'expérience de l'Orient chrétien des premiers siècles,* Paris 1992; *Therapeutique des maladies spirituelles. Une introduction à la tradition ascetique de l'Eglise orthodoxe,* Paris 1997; *La divinisation de l'homme selon saint Maxime le Confesseur,* Paris 1996; *Ceci est mon corps. Le sens chrétien du corps selon les Pères de l'Eglise,* Geneva 1996; *Pour une éthique de la procréation. Éléments d'anthropologie patristique,* Paris 1998.

Address: 14 rue des Alouettes, 57350 Spicheren, France.

PATRICK DONDELINGER was born in Luxembourg in 1966 and studied in Luxembourg and Paris; he has doctorates in the history of religions and religious anthropology, and in theology. He teaches the anthropology of rites at the Institut Supérieur de Liturgie of the Institut Catholique in Paris and directs research at the Inderdisciplinary Institute for Psychology and Psychohygiene at Freiburg in Breisgau. His thesis on 'The Exorcism of the Possessed according to the Roman Ritual and its Ecclesial Interpretation in the Contemporary West' will shortly be published in Paris.

Address: Institut Supérieur de Liturgie, Institut Catholique de Paris, 21, rue d Assas, F 75270 Paris Cedex 06, France.

EUGEN BISER was born in 1918. Between 1965 and 1973 he was Professor of Fundamental Theology in Passau and Würzburg, and between 1974 and 1986 Professor of Christian Thought and Philosophy of Religion in Munich; since 1987 he has been Dean of Class 8 of the European Academy, Salzburg. His most recent publications are: *Des Glaubens geschichtliche Wende*, Graz 1986; *Glaubensprognose*, Graz 1991; *Paulus: Zeuge und Mystike*, Munich 1991; *Der Mensch des uneingelösten Versprechen*, Düsseldorf 1993; *Überwindung des Lebensangst*, Munich 1996; *Einweisung ins Christentum*, Düsseldorf 1997.

Address: Seniorenstudium der LMU, Veterinärstrasse 1, D–80539 Munich, Germany.

GISBERT GRESHAKE was born in 1933 in Recklinghausen, Westphalia; he gained licentiates in philosophy and theology in Rome and a doctorate in theology in Münster. He was ordained priest in 1960 and engaged in pastoral work for many years. After his Habilitation at Tübingen in 1972, from 1974 to 1985 he was Professor of Dogmatic Theology und the History of Dogma in Vienna; since 1985 he has been Professor of Dogmatics and Ecumenics in Freiburg im Breisgau. He is co-editor of *Fontes Christianae*, and technical advisor to the *Lexikon für Theologie und Kirche*. He has written around 30 articles and 400 articles, above all on questions of spiritual theology, eschatology, and the doctrines of grace and the Trinity. His most recent book is *Der dreieine Gott*, Freiburg [3]1998.

Address: Albert-Ludwigs-Universität, Institut für systematische Theologie, Postfach 79085, Freiburg, Germany.

KRISTIAAN DEPOORTERE was born in 1946. He is Professor of Pastoral Theology at the Catholic University of Leuven and Professor of Sacramental Theology at the Theological Centre of the Archdiocese of Mechelen-Brussels. His most recent publications are *A Different God. A*

Christian View of Suffering, Leuven and Grand Rapids 1995; *Qui es-tu Jésus?*, Brussels and Namur 1997.

MATTHEW SCHOFFELEERS was born at Beek, in the Dutch province of Limburg, in 1928. He studied theology at the Montfortian Seminary of Oirschot, where he was ordained priest. He obtained a doctorate in Social Anthropology at Oxford, and worked for some twenty years as a rural missionary and university teacher in Malawi. Following this, he taught Anthropology of Religion at the Free University, Amsterdam, and at the University of Utrecht. He is now emeritus professor. His books include: *Guardians of the Land. Essays on Central African Territorial Cults*, Zimbabwe 1978, and *River of Blood. The Genesis of a Martyr Cult in Southern Malawi. c. AD. 1600*, Madison, Wisconsin 1992. He has written many articles.

Address: Apollolaan 634, 2324 CK Leiden, The Netherlands.

ELIZA KUPPOZHACKEL is a member of the International Congregation of the Medical Mission Sisters. She has a Masters Degree in Social Work and an MD in Alternative Medicine, and is well trained in oriental medicine, yoga and several non-drug therapies. She has taken the initiative in starting several innovative programmes to promote a new health culture through a holistic and integrated approach to health. For the last ten years she has been the course director of Ayushya, a centre for healing and integration, and is also the founder Chairperson of the Pranic Healing Foundation of Kerala and the Vice-President of the Voluntary Health Association of India. She has compiled and edited a book on herbal medicine and home remedies and has contributed many articles to national and international publications.

Address: Medical Mission Sisters – USHUS, Collectorate PO, Kottayam 686002, Kerala State, India.

ANNETH NYAGAWA MUNGA is a priest within the Evangelical Lutheran Church in Tanzania. In May 1998 she completed her doctoral studies in Systematic Theology at the University of Lund, Sweden. Her thesis is titled 'Uamsho. A Theological Study of the Proclamation of the Revival Movement within the Evangelical Lutheran Church in Tanzania'. She is living temporarily in Sweden but expects to return to Tanzania in the near future.

Address: Lund University, Department of Theology and Religious Studies, Allhelgona Kyrkogata 8, S–223 62 Lund, Sweden.

Concilium 1998/5: Illness and Healing

The editors wish to thank the great number of colleagues who contributed in a most helpful way to the Final Project.

R. Aguirre	Bilbao	Spain
P. Baud	Pully	Switzerland
E. Barbieri Massini	Rome	Italy
T. Berger	North Carolina	USA
M. A. O Brien	Box Hill	Australia
C. Carozzo	Genoa	Italy
G. Cereti	Rome	Italy
P. de Clerck	Paris	France
J. Coleman	Los Angeles	USA
V. Conzemius	Lucerne	Switzerland
H. Czosnyka	Saint Louis	USA
J. H. Erickson	Crestwood	USA
E. Farrugia	Rome	Italy
C. Floristan	Madrid	Spain
R. Gibellini	Brescia	Italy
T. J. Green	Washington	USA
B. van Iersel	Nijmegen	Netherlands
M. Klöckener	Fribourg	Switzerland
M. Lamberigts	Leuven	Belgium
A. Lampe	Chemutal-Quintana	Mexico
H. Laubach	Mainz	Germany
G. Lukken	Tilburg	Netherlands
S. McEvenue	Montreal	Canada
A. Melloni	Reggio Emilia	Italy
N. Mette	Münster	Germany
C. Méroz	Neuchâtel	Switzerland
R. Modras	Saint Louis	USA
E. Pace	Padua	Italy
S. Painadath	Kerala	India
O. H. Pesch	Hamburg	Germany
P. Philibert	Notre Dame	USA
D. N. Power	Washington	USA
H. Raguer	Montserrat	Spain
A. Skowronek	Warsaw	Poland
C. Soetens	Brussels	Belgium
C. Theobald	Paris	France
R. Torfs	Leuven	Belgium
M. Vidal	Madrid	Spain

Concilium 1990-1999

1990

1   On the Threshold of the Third Millennium   *The Concilium Foundation*
2   The Ethics of World Religions and Human Rights   *Hans Küng and Jürgen Moltmann*
3   Asking and Thanking   *Christian Duquoc and Casiano Floristan*
4   Collegiality put to the Test   *James Provost and Knut Walf*
5   Coping with Failure   *Norbert Greinacher and Norbert Mette*
6   1492-1992: The Voice of the Victims   *Leonardo Boff and Virgil Elizondo*

1991

1   The Bible and Its Readers   *Wim Beuken, Sean Freyne and Anton Weiler*
2   The Pastoral Care of the Sick   *Mary Collins and David Power*
3   Aging   *Lisa Sowle Cahill and Dietmar Mieth*
4   No Heaven without Earth   *Johann Baptist Metz and Edward Schillebeeckx*
5   *Rerum Novarum*: 100 Years of Catholic Social Teaching   *Gregory Baum
     and John Coleman*
6   The Special Nature of Women   *Anne Carr and Elisabeth Schüssler Fiorenza*

1992

1   Towards the African Synod   *Giuseppe Alberigo and Alphonse Ngindu Mushete*
2   The New Europe   *Norbert Greinacher and Norbert Mette*
3   Fundamentalism as an Ecumenical Challenge   *Hans Küng and Jürgen Moltmann*
4   Where is God?   *Christian Duquoc and Casiano Floristan*
5   The Tabu of Democracy in the Church   *James Provost and Knut Walf*
6   The Debate on Modernity   *Claude Geffré and Jean-Pierre Jossua*

1993

1   Messianism through History   *Wim Beuken and Anton Weiler*
2   Any Room for Christ in Asia?   *Leonardo Boff and Virgil Elizondo*
3   The Spectre of Mass Death   *David Power and Kabasele Lumbala*
4   Migrants and Refugees   *Dietmar Mieth and Lisa Sowle Cahill*
5   Reincarnation or Resurrection?   *Hermann Häring and Johann Baptist Metz*
6   Mass Media   *John Coleman and Miklós Tomka*

1994

1   Violence against Women   *Elisabeth Schüssler Fiorenza and Mary Shawn Copeland*
2   Christianity and Cultures   *Norbert Greinacher and Norbert Mette*
3   Islam: A Challenge for Christianity   *Hans Küng and Jürgen Moltmann*
4   Mysticism and the Institutional Crisis   *Christian Duquoc and Gustavo Gutiérrez*
5   Catholic Identity   *James Provost and Knut Walf*
6   Why Theology?   *Claude Geffré and Werner Jeanrond*

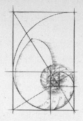

John Templeton Foundation

1999

Call for Exemplary Papers on Humility in Theology

To encourage scholarly research on matters of both spiritual and scientific significance, the John Templeton Foundation invites scholars to submit published papers on topics regarding the constructive interaction of:

- Theology and the natural sciences
- Religion and the medical sciences, or
- Religion and the behavioral sciences.

These papers must proceed from professional scholarship and display a spirit of intellectual humility, a respect for varied theological traditions, and an attitude of open-minded inquiry into the varied ways in which theology/religion and the empirical sciences can be mutually informative. Papers must have been published or accepted for publication in a peer-reviewed journal or similarly selective scholarly publication, be between 3,000 and 10,000 words in length, and be accompanied by a 600-word précis (in English, even if the paper is not).

Prizes ranging from $500 to $3000 will be awarded in November 1999. The deadline for submission of papers is June 1, 1999.

For full details and application forms, please visit our web site, or write to:
Exemplary Papers Program Director, **John Templeton Foundation**
Five Radnor Corporate Center, Suite 100 ▪ 100 Matsonford Road
Radnor, Pennsylvania 19087-8322 USA
www.templeton.org

Reference: CON

Concilium Subscription Information - outside North America

Individual Annual Subscription (five issues): £25.00

Institution Annual Subscription (five issues): £35.00

Airmail subscriptions: add £10.00

Individual issues: £8.95 each

New subscribers please return this form:
for a two-year subscription, double the appropriate rate

(for individuals)   £25.00   (1/2 years)   . . . .

(for institutions)   £35.00   (1/2 years)   . . . .

Airmail postage
outside Europe +£10.00   (1/2 years)   . . . .

                            Total . . . .

I wish to subscribe for one/two years as an individual/institution
(delete as appropriate)

Name/Institution . . . .

Address . . . .

. . . .

. . . .

I enclose a cheque for . . . . payable to SCM Press Ltd

Please charge my Access/Visa/Mastercard no. . . . .

Signature . . . . .Expiry Date . . . .

Please return this form to:
SCM PRESS LTD   9 - 17 St Albans Place   London   N1 0NX